The Authors

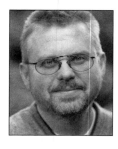

Hans-Ulrich Hecker, M.D.
Medical specialist in general medicine, acu-
puncture, naturopathy, and homeopathy.
Lecturer in Naturopathy and Acupuncture,
University of Schleswig-Holstein, Germany.
Research Director of Education in Natur-
opathy and Acupuncture, Academy of Con-
tinuing Medical Education of the Regional
Medical Association of Schleswig-Holstein.
Certified Medical Quality Manager.
Assessor of the European Foundation of Quality Management
(EFQM).
e-mail:praxis@go3docs.de
www.go3docs.de

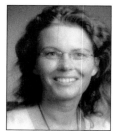

Angelika Steveling, M.D.
Chiropractor,
NLP practitioner.
Head of the Department of Traditional
Medicine at the Institute for Radiology and
Microtherapy, University of Witten-
Herdecke, Germany.
Lecturer for Acupuncture Continuing Edu-
cation, Regional Medical Associations of Schleswig-Holstein and
Westphalia-Lippe.
Lecturer of the German Society of Physicians for Acupuncture
(DÄGFA).
e-mail: info@akupunktur-ruhr.de
www.akupunktur-ruhr.de

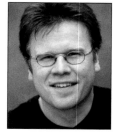

Elmar T. Peuker, M.D.
Medical specialist in general medicine,
anatomy, chiropractic, and naturopathy.
Lecturer for Acupuncture and Naturopathy
Continuing Education, Regional Medical
Association of Schleswig-Holstein. Diploma
in Health Economy.
Head of the Complementary Medicine
Study Group, Department of Anatomy, Wilhelm University of
Westphalia, Muenster, Germany.
Lecturer at the British Medical Acupuncture Society (BMAS), UK.
e-mail:info@integrative-medizin.de
www.integrative-medizin.de

For contributors please see page VI.

Microsystems Acupuncture
The Complete Guide:
Ear—Scalp—Mouth—Hand

Hans Ulrich Hecker, M.D., L.Ac.
Physician in Private Practice
Kiel, Germany

Elmar Peuker, M.D., L.Ac.
Clinical Anatomist
Physician in Private Practice
Muenster, Germany

Angelika Steveling, M.D., L.Ac.
Physician in Private Practice
Essen, Germany

With contributions by
Michaela Bijak, John Blank, Timm J. Filler, Hans Garten, Jochen Gleditsch,
Bernhard Lichtenauer, Kay Liebchen, Dieter Muehlhoff, Helmut Nissel,
Rudolf Rauch, Karen Spiegel, Daniela Stockenhuber, Karsten Strauss,
Beate Strittmatter, Max Wiesner-Zechmeister

344 illustrations

Thieme
Stuttgart · New York

Library of Congress Cataloging-in-Publication Data

Hecker, Hans-Ulrich.
[Lehrbuch und Repetitorium, Ohr-, Schaedel-,
Mund-Hand–Akupunktur. English]
Microsystems acupuncture : the complete guide :
ear–scalp–mouth–hand / Hans Ulrich Hecker,
Elmar Peuker, Angelika Steveling ;
with contributions by Michaela Bijak ... [et al.] ;
translated by Angela Trowell.
    p. ; cm.
Authorized and rev. translation of: Lehrbuch und
Repetitorium, Ohr-, Schaedel-, Mund-
Hand–Akupunktur. 3rd ed. 2002.
Includes bibliographical references and index.
ISBN 3-13-129111-7 (GTV : alk. paper) –
ISBN 1-58890-329-X (TNY : alk. paper)
1. Acupuncture points. 2. Acupuncture.
I. Peuker, Elmar T. II. Steveling, Angelika. III. Title.
[DNLM: 1. Acupuncture Therapy–instrumentation.
2. Acupuncture Therapy–methods. 3. Hand.
4. Head. WB 369 H449L 2006a]
RM184.5.H43 2006
615.8'92–dc22   2005023525

This book is an authorized, revised, and expanded
translation of the 3rd German edition published
and copyrighted 2002 by Hipprokates Verlag,
Stuttgart, Germany. Title of the German edition:
Lehrbuch und Repetitorium. Ohr-, Schaedel-,
Mund-, Hand- Akupunktur. Behandlung ueber das
Somatotop

Translator: Angela M. J. Trowell, Granada, Spain

© 2006 Georg Thieme Verlag,
Rüdigerstrasse 14, 70469 Stuttgart, Germany
http://www.thieme.de
Thieme New York, 333 Seventh Avenue,
New York, NY 10001 USA
http://www.thieme.com

Typesetting by Martin Wunderlich, Kiel
Printed in Germany by Appl, Wemding

ISBN 3-13-129111-7 (GTV)
ISBN 1-58890-329-X (TNY)   1 2 3 4 5 6

Preface

For the first time a book has been published which discusses all of the relevant microsystems of acupuncture in practice today. In addition to ear acupuncture, where both Western schools according to Nogier and Bahr as well as Chinese schools are considered, special chapters are given to the following; Chinese Scalp Acupuncture, Yamamoto New Scalp Acupuncture, Mouth Acupuncture, Chinese Hand Acupuncture, Korean Hand Acupuncture, and New Point-Based Pain and Organ Therapy. In addition, the use of laser acupuncture and addiction treatment used with acupuncture is also considered.

The proven team of editors of the *Color Atlas of Acupuncture* and *Practice of Acupuncture* has been successful in gaining international recognition as acupuncture specialists through this book. The authors who have contributed to this book have been active in the field of acupuncture training for many years across various disciplines. In many cases, they also teach in universities as lecturers or heads of institutes. *Microsystems Acupuncture* highlights the most recent views on the diagnoses and therapies used for different somatotopies. The didactical concept, which has been developed by the team of editors and proven in practice, is a guarantee for your learning success.

We would like to thank all of our colleagues who were involved in this book project. We thank Axel Nikolaus for the photographic conversion and Mr Wunderlich for the graphic organization. Last but not least, we give special thanks to our editor, Angelika-Marie Findgott, whose wealth of experience and linguistic authority made the translation and update of this standard textbook possible.

Hans-Ulrich Hecker
Angelika Steveling
Elmar T. Peuker

Contributors

Michaela Bijak
Physician in Private Practice
Vienna, Austria

John Blank
Portland Alternative Health Center
Portland, OR, USA

Timm J. Filler
Professor
Clinical Anatomist
Head of the Clinical Anatomy Division
University of Muenster
Muenster, Germany

Hans Garten
Anesthesiologist
Physician in Private Practice
Munich, Germany

Jochen Gleditsch
Otolaryngologist, Dentist
Honorary President of the German Medical
Acupuncture Association
Baierbrunn, Germany

Bernhard Lichtenauer
Physician in Private Practice
Schwarzau, Austria

Kay Liebchen
Orthopedist, Rheumatologist
Physician in Private Practice
Schleswig, Germany

Dieter Muehlhoff
Oncologist, Naturopath
Physician in Private Practice
Felde, Germany

Helmut Nissel
Professor
Director of the Kaiserin-Elisabeth-Hospital Vienna
Vienna, Austria

Rudolf Rauch
Physician in Private Practice
Vienna, Austria

Karen Spiegel
Naturopath, Physician in Private Practice
Kiel, Germany

Daniela Stockenhuber
Physician in Private Practice
Purkersdorf, Austria

Karsten Strauss
Addiction Therapist
Institute for Addiction Medicine
Barkelsby, Germany

Beate Strittmatter
Naturopath, Sports medicine
Physician in Private Practice
Spiesen-Elversberg, Germany

Max Wiesner-Zechmeister
Physician in Private Practice
Ried, Austria

Content

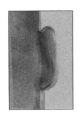

1 Basic Principles of Auricular Acupuncture (Page 1)

H.-U. Hecker, A. Steveling, E.T. Peuker, B. Strittmatter, T.J. Filler

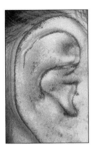

2 Topography and Indications of Auricular Acupuncture Points According to Regions (Page 37)

H.-U. Hecker, B. Strittmatter, A. Steveling, E.T. Peuker

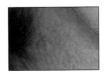

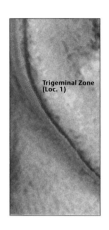

3 Treatment of Major Illnesses
(Page 129)
H.-U. Hecker, D. Mühlhoff,
A. Steveling, E.T. Peuker,
K.-H. Junghanns †

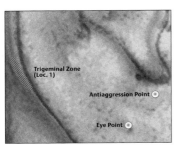

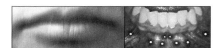
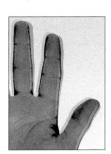

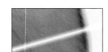

Microsystems Acupuncture Today
(J. Gleditsch)

Various Microsystems: Historical Background

Traditional Chinese Medicine (TCM) during the past 50 years has been supplemented and amplified by a new form of acupuncture called microsystem acupuncture.

Microsystem acupuncture is based on particular somatotopic fields comprising specific points of correspondence. Such somatotopic fields were mainly discovered in the West. Microsystems are situated on circumscribed parts of the body, for example, the auricle, the scalp, and the oral cavity. As microsystems resemble cartographies of the organism, they have an allusion to the somatotopic homunculus, as represented at the cerebral hemispheres.

Each of the microsystem points has a clearly defined correlation to, and interrelation with, a particular organ or function. Thus, microsystem acupuncture is a very effective treatment and is established for diagnosis as well.

The first microsystem to be discovered in the early 1950's was the system of specific points on the auricle. It was the French doctor *Nogier* who decoded the functional correspondences of the respective auricular points. This punctual cartography resembles a replica of an upside-down embryo. The auricular microsystem is very detailed even though the specific points are densely packed.

Ear acupuncture was continuously refined by *Nogier* himself as well as by Chinese and Russian schools of acupuncture. Nowadays, auriculotherapy is acknowledged and has gained acceptance worldwide, owing to its therapeutic and diagnostic qualities.

It may be recalled that as early as the close of the 19th century, foot reflexology—probably of Native American Indian origin—had been rediscovered in the U.S.

In the same period, *Fliess* of Berlin found out that certain digestive, urogenital as well as respiratory disorders responded well when he swabbed specific endonasal zones with a cocaine solution. Obviously, the respective areas of lower and middle nasal conchae were inter-related with specific internal organs and functions. Nasal reflex therapy using specific zones of the nasal mucous membrane was then widely accepted and used by many European practitioners.

Together with auriculotherapy, Yamamoto's New Scalp Acupuncture (YNSA) has become a very popular form of microsystem acupuncture. In the 1970's *Toshikatsu Yamamoto* of Japan discovered various somatotopic zones on the scalp. Specific "basic" zones represent functions of the locomotor system and of the sense organs. In addition, specific "Y"-zones, of 12 points each, represent the respective main channels of TCM. Both basic and Y-zones, as found in the frontal/temporal area, are mirrored once more in the occipital region. Originally, Dr. *Yamamoto* had discovered striking inter-correlations between the traditional Japanese diagnostic zones of the abdominal wall and specific temporal points. Pain sensitivity and induration of a particular abdominal site is indicative of dysregulation of one of the TCM channels. Therapy applied to a Y-point brings about an immediate dispersal of the corresponding abdominal induration.

Oral acupuncture, also discovered in the 1970's, is another form of microsystem acupuncture. Intercorrelations of the enoral acupoints are identical with those of the five groups of teeth, as decoded by *Voll* by means of electro-acupuncture as early as 1965. One particular meridian couple is represented in each one of five dental groups as well as in the adjacent acupoints. In addition to these vestibular points, there are retromolar points, situated beyond the wisdom teeth. These retromolar points are very effective when treating dysfunctions of the locomotor system.

Hand acupuncture has proved to be another effective form of microsystem therapy. During the last decades, Korean Su-Yok ("hand–foot") acupuncture has become popular in Western countries. In Korean hand acupuncture, the twelve channels as well as reflex points of inner organs and functions and of the skeletal structure are represented by a multitude of points on the palmar and dorsal sides of the hand. A Chinese variant of hand acupuncture provides specific points which are rather related to various indications, with no apparent systematic cartography.

Finally, a somatotopic system situated at the lower leg and foot, discovered by *Siener* of Germany, has proved effective in therapy.

Characteristics Common to All Microsystems

Common features of microsystem points are: the totality of points comprised in a particular micro-acu-point system (MAPS) constitutes a functional image of the whole organism in a clearly defined partial area. The respective microsystem points are representative of particular organs and functions and/or of channels of TCM. In this way, microsystem points function as distant points; they always provide treatment, even if a site of pain or dysfunction is not accessible locally. Effects triggered via specific microsystem points are reproducible effects.

After several decades of practice and experience, it has become evident that microsystem therapy works differently to TCM. While the meridian points, owing to the non-stop *qi* circulation, are constantly available for therapy, in microsystem therapy an "on/off" mechanism is obvious. This results in microsystem points being strictly reactive. They are detectable only in the case of a functional disturbance of the correlated organ. Thus microsystem points show up like "warning signals."

The activation of microsystem points results in a measurable change of electrical conductivity. This enables bio-electrical point detection. In addition, activated microsystem points are clearly tender to pressure as a rule.

Experience shows that functional disorders are naturally "signaled" simultaneously to analogous points of all microsystems. The degree of point activation, however, may vary from one microsystem to the other. Treatment can be optimized by not sticking to one microsystem only, but by

including analogous points of other microsystems as well.

As a rule, if an active point of one microsystem has been treated successfully, this results in analogous points of the other microsystems being deactivated—"deleted"—instantly. Analogous points cease to be detectable.

The "deleting" or "extinguishing" phenomenon indicates a) that a positive therapeutic impulse has been triggered, b) that the choice of points was obviously beneficial, and c) that the patient responds well to acupuncture.

The synonymous terms microsystems, micro-acu-point systems (MAPS), or somatotopic acupuncture are applicable to each of the following variants:

► Systems offering a basically complete organotropic representation of the organism via points or areas of correspondence (e.g. on the auricle, on the soles of the feet).

► Systems offering mini-scale representations of the channels depicting every one of the points in a very condensed space (e.g. Korean hand acupuncture).

► Systems offering a 12-point representation of the 12 main channels (e.g. YNSA, scalp acupuncture).

► Systems offering punctual representation of the respective coupled channel pairs, that is, of the five functional networks ("elements" of TCM), for example, oral acupuncture.

Incomplete micro-point systems specialized in a selection of indications (e.g. nasal reflex zones, Chinese hand acupuncture).

Interestingly, the back *shu* points, which are representative of the 12 channels, also meet these conditions. In this way, they form a link between TCM and microsystem acupuncture.

The therapeutic effects of acupuncture have been scientifically proven. This applies in particular to pain management achieved by pain research in recent decades. Modulation mechanisms involving endorphin and transmitter activation explain the analgesic effect of both meridian and microsystem acupuncture points. Moreover, spasmolytic, antiphlogistic, sedative, and immunomodulating effects indicate involvement of the autonomic nervous system. According to *Bossy*, a neuroanatomist at the University of Nîmes, France, it is the reticular formation, where the afferences from the organ in question meet the microsystem point stimuli.

In clinical studies conducted by universities, microsystem points have proved to be superior, particularly on account of their immediate effect, especially in treating locomotor disorders.

Phenomena as seen in microsystem acupuncture may be interpreted in terms of cybernetics and system theory; this applies particularly to mutual networking as well as to the "deleting" phenomenon.

As is known today, the volumes of information, their complexity and networking are increasing in open dissipative systems. An increase in information implies an increase in order. Thus, properties which did not exist previously may emerge, as is the case with nonlinear systems. Fractal geometry, as inaugurated by *Mandelbrot*, works in the field of nonlinear equations and complex numbers. The recurrence of self-emulating figures is striking when the vast variety of forms is being scaled down progressively. The principle of fractalization (i.e. the similarity principle) has been recognized as the fundamental feature of self-organization in nature. The modern fractal-field model of organism structure opens the way to an understanding of the appearance, structure, and activity of microacupuncture systems.

In living systems, fractalization leads to organisms creating a number of quantum copies of themselves. These replicas seem to provide information exchange between the inner organs and the environment. In terms of cybernetics, therefore, microacupuncture systems are homeostats. The biological significance of these multiple copies is to guarantee greater internal stability and regulation resources.

1 Basic Principles of Auricular Acupuncture

(H.-U. Hecker, A. Steveling,
E.T. Peuker, B. Strittmatter, T.J. Filler)

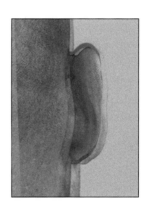

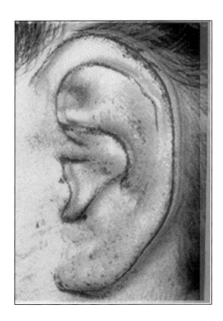

Introduction

Auricular acupuncture represents a special form of acupuncture and is often used as a complement to body acupuncture.

It is based on a self-contained model of thought. A core idea is the concept of somatopy. This expression is composed of the Greek words soma (= body) and topos (= location) and means the differentiated mapping of the body in one area (here the auricula). Often the term microsystem is used synonymously, although strictly speaking this includes the whole diagnostic and therapeutic concept. Somatopies are familiar from different parts of the central nervous system, for example locomotor somatopy in the Gyrus precentralis or sensory somatopy in the Gyrus postcentralis. By means of somatopy, corresponding constructs are also found for other senses, such as tonotopy for hearing and retinotopy for sight.

As a rule, somatopic assignments are not relative to the size of the mapped region but in accordance with the expression of the respective qualities. Thus, in some cases in the central projection areas there are grotesquely disproportionate representations of the body that are often referred to as homunculus. It is a similar story for the familiar microsystems. The representation of the body on the ear vaguely calls to mind an inverted fetus, the proportions and location of which vary considerably, however, depending on the school of auricular acupuncture (see below).

Unlike body acupuncture, the points on the auricula are only irritated and thus identifiable if there is a disturbance in the respective region of the body of which they are a representative projection. This basic principle also applies to the other microsystem zones.

Therapeutic procedures involving the auricula have been mentioned since antiquity. Thus, Hippocrates is said to have tried to cure impotence by means of bloodletting from the outer ear; Egyptian sailors are said to have tried to improve their sight for navigation by pricking their ear lobes (among other things, the Eye Point in the modern auriculotherapy model is also found in the ear lobe).

Time and time again, cauterization of the auricula was undertaken as a therapy for sciatic pain. We know of corresponding applications by, for example, Persian healers. But in Western Europe there are also references to such therapeutic approaches. Thus, as far back as 1637, *Zactus Lusitanus* described cauterization of the ear as a therapy for sciatic pain in Portugal; in 1810 *Ignaz Colla* described cauterization of the rear side of the auricula for the same reason. In 1717, *Valsalva* treated toothache via the auricula. In the second part (*Ling Shu*) of the *Huang Di Nei Jing*, there are observations regarding treatment in the area around the auricula. However, beyond this there are no references to a concept of auricular acupuncture by the standard authors of Chinese medicine.

As early as the 18th century, numerous publications reported the benefits of cauterization of the auricula as a therapy for sciatica. However, it was not until 1950 that the French neurologist *Paul Nogier* attempted to write a comprehensive description of the therapy of the auricula. He discovered cauterization marks on the anthelix in numerous patients who had been treated by a healer (Mme. *Barrin*) for sciatic pain. The patients reported astonishing success with this therapy, leading *Nogier* to further investigate the phenomenon. He also began his own trials with cauterization but then turned to "less barbaric" methods such as pricking with needles or pins, with which he achieved equally good results. He came to the conclusion that disturbances of the body (over and above sciatic pain) could be demonstrated on a regular basis by means of sensitive or painful points on the auricula. He interpreted the representation of the body on the auricula as the image of an inverted fetus—he was thus able to assign the point on the antihelix usually used for sciatic pain therapy the representation zone L4.

In February 1956, at the invitation of the famous acupuncturist *Niboyet*, *Nogier* presented his findings at the first congress of the Société méditerranéenne d'Acupuncture in Marseilles, France. At the instance of *Gerhard Bachmann* (then Chairman of the Deutsche Gesellschaft für Akupunktur [German Society for Acupuncture]), these findings were published in the *Deutsche Zeitschrift für Akupunktur* (German Acupuncture Journal) in 1957. The findings were not known about in China until the beginning of 1959. Here, although in the past the auricula had been regarded as an important topographical region at which some meridians of body acupuncture meet, independent auricular acupuncture had not previously existed. It was not until the end of 1959 that the expression auricular acupuncture (*er zhen*) first appeared in Chinese acupuncture literature. Subsequently, "Chinese auricular acupuncture" developed with its own nomenclature and mapping of the ear points which in Europe was employed and interpreted by *König* and *Wancura* using a numeric system. Less and less mention is made of the basis of this Chinese auricular acupuncture (the findings of *Paul Nogier*) in more recent Chinese tutorials.

Nor are there any references in the classic works of Chinese medicine to the microsystems prevalent to a greater or lesser degree in diagnosis and therapy. As a rule, all theories about microsystems are a few years to decades old and have in some cases been implemented retrospectively in one or more of the systems of Chinese medicine.

Taking as a basis the publication of the findings of *Paul Nogier* in the *Deutsche Zeitschrift für Akupunktur*, translations or abstracts were also published in Japan, what was then Ceylon (today's Sri Lanka), and the former USSR.

Today there are several schools of auricular acupuncture; besides the establishment of schools based on *Nogier* and *Bahr* on the one hand, and the Chinese school on the other, there has been increasing research activity by Russian scientists based on *R.A. Durinjan* and *F.G. Portnov*.

The slight variations in point localizations and approaches in diagnosis and therapy which exist in part between the different schools must not be regarded as rivaling each other, but rather interpreted on the basis of the respective model and the practical approach. Thus, in part, Chinese points represent functional relationships, the *Nogier* points rather the anatomical correlative. Lastly, a careful investigative technique is crucial for auricular acupuncture in order to identify the individually active points and thus be able to employ them for therapy.

In this book, both the common laws and the differences in the localization of points are described and interpreted, providing the therapist with alternatives which upon closer examination prove to be an enrichment of the range of therapies.

Basic Principles of Auricular Acupuncture

Basic Principles

Anatomy of the Outer Ear (Auricula)

The outer ear together with the auditory canal forms the auricula. Its shape corresponds to the underlying elastic cartilage close to the skin. Only the ear lobe contains no cartilage. Over the dorsomedial area, the skin of the auricula is thin and can be moved relatively easily with regard to the perichondrium. Anterolaterally, the skin is firm and relatively difficult to move.

Both external muscles and own muscles are attached to the auricula. The external muscles permit some people to obtain residual movement of the ear and form part of the mimetic musculature. The ear's own muscles correspond to the remains of a sphincter system with which the auditory canal can be closed in animals which live in water or underground.

Although the individual internal shape of the ear may vary greatly (and also when the two sides are compared), there are some anatomical landmarks which are relatively constant and can thus serve as reference points for locating the acupuncture points of the ear.

The outer shape of the auricula is formed by the helical rim (helix). The helix originates on the floor of the concha and ascends as the root of helix (crus of helix). It is followed by the body of the helix which descends as the tail of the helix toward the ear lobe. The helix then turns into the ear lobe (auricular lobule). In the upper, rear part of the helix, we usually find a protrusion or widening of the helical rim, the helical tubercle (Darwinian tubercle), which corresponds to the tip of some mammals' ears. The anthelix runs parallel to the helix. It originates in the upper part of the auricula with two legs, the inferior anthelical crus and the superior anthelical crus. Between the two anthelical crura lies the triangular fossa. The anthelix turns into the antitragus in the lower part of the ear. The border between them is formed by the postantitragal fossa.

Between the helix and the superior anthelical crus plus anthelix lies the scapha.

The tragus is bordered by the intertragic notch to the antitragus and the supratragic notch to the crus of helix. At the bottom of the auricula lies the cavity of concha. The concha is divided by the ascending crus of helix into two parts, the superior concha (cymba) and the inferior concha. The outer auditory canal lies in the inferior concha and is covered from view by the tragus.

The anatomical landmarks of the outside of the auricula partly find their correlate on the rear side. Thus, on the dorsal side of the auricula the helical rim and the eminence of scapha of the sulcus anthelicis can be directly delimited medially. Dorsally both parts of the cavity of concha become the superior and inferior eminence of concha, which are often separated from each other by a sulcus posterior centralis. The equivalents of the crura anthelices (as sulci) and the triangular fossa (as eminentia) on the dorsal side can less frequently be delimited so clearly.

The usually biconcave reverse side of the ear lobe is called the fovea retrobularis.

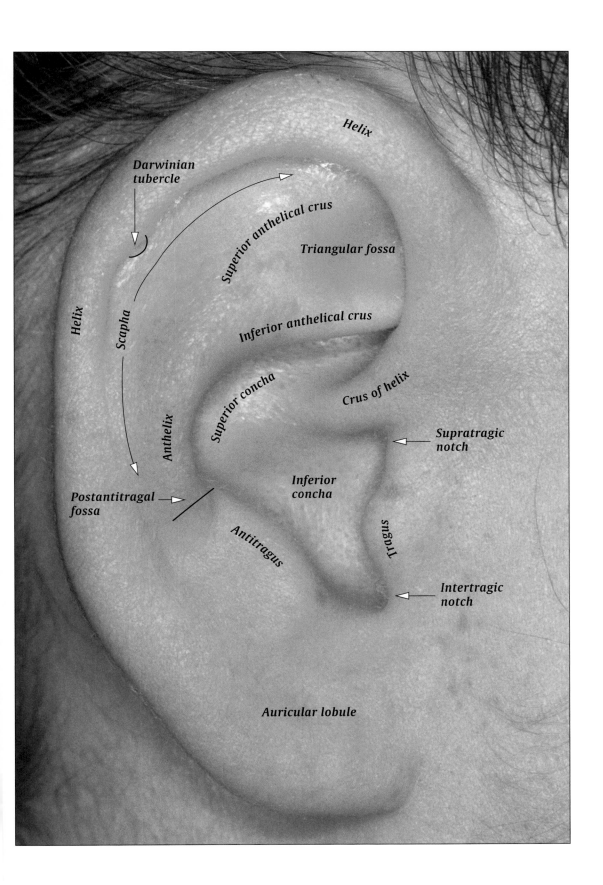

Zones of Auricular Innervation and Embryological Assignment According to *Nogier*

Although *Nogier* did not carry out any anatomical or embryological investigations of his own, several assignments can be found in his records, usually with reference to the research done by *Valsalva*. According to this, the auricula is innervated by three nerves:

- ► The auricular branch of the vagus nerve

- ► The auriculotemporal nerve of the trigeminal nerve

- ► The great auricular nerve of the cervical plexus.

The auricular branch of the vagus nerve innervates the concha. According to this concept, the "entodermal" organs are projected here.

The great auricular nerve of the cervical plexus supplies the lobule, the outer helical rim up to approximately the Darwinian tubercle, and the back of the ear. These areas correspond to organs in the ectodermal germ layer. The remaining, and by far the largest, part of the ear is innervated by the auriculotemporal nerve of the trigeminal nerve. The mesodermal organs are projected here.

According to *Nogier*, the different zones are assigned to different functional areas:

Entodermal zone	►	Metabolism, organs
Mesodermal zone	►	Motor system
Ectodermal zone	►	Head and central nervous system

In line with this tripartition, *Nogier* found one control point for each functional area; these are the Omega Points.

Auriculotemporal nerve
(trigeminal nerve)

Auricular branch
(vagus nerve)

Great auricular nerve
(cervical plexus)

Zones of Auricular Innervation According to *Nogier*

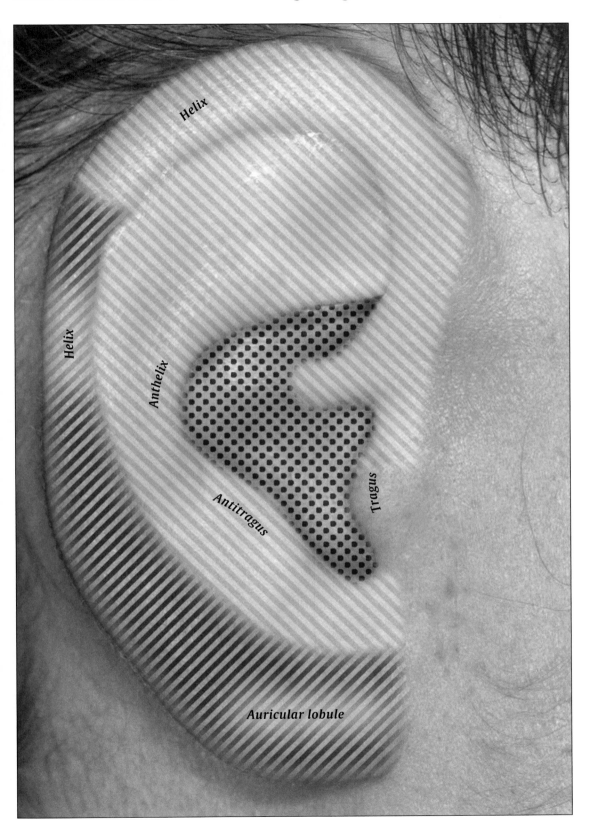

Zones of Auricular Innervation According to *R.A. Durinjan*

The description of the auricular zones of innervation and the various somatopic representations according to the Russian school goes back to *R.A. Durinjan*. The first comprehensive German-language presentation of Russian auriculotherapy came from *R. Umlauf* and was published in 1988 in the *German Journal of Acupuncture* (Deutsche Zeitschrift für Akupunktur).

According to *Durinjan*, the following five nerves participate in the innervation of the auricula:

► Fibers of the cervical plexus,

► The trigeminal nerve,

► The intermediate nerve of the facial nerve,

► The glossopharyngeal nerve,

► The auricular branch of the vagus nerve.

The innervation zones show distinct overlaps of all the areas innervated by the five participating nerves. No auricular zone is therefore exclusively innervated by one single nerve. This might explain why two or more acupuncture points of different functions are projected on identical anatomical sites. Likewise, projections of the same organ are ascribed to different sites of localization. For example, we find projections which correspond to the parenchyma of the organ, next to them projections of the corresponding nervous innervation, and, finally, projections representing the functional state of the organ. Due to the variation in auricular shape, it is conceivable that the overlaps of innervation zones also vary individually. Thus, the frequently described points are really zones rather than points in which the actual ear acupuncture point must be searched for according to individual circumstances. No doubt, this approach goes back to *Nogier*, who tried to find individual representations of acupuncture points by means of the auriculocardiac reflex (ACR) (cf. p. 30).

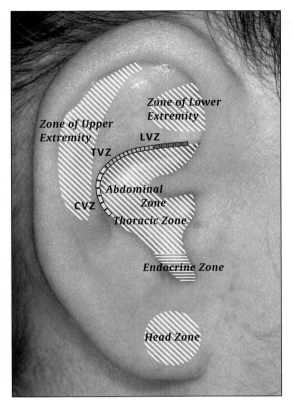

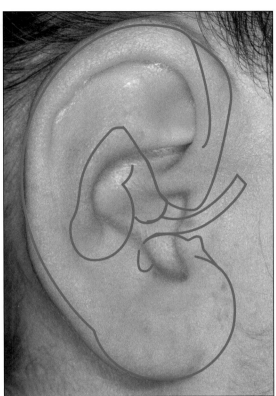

Localization of organs and extremities according to the inverted fetus model.

Projection of the Skeleton According to *Nogier*

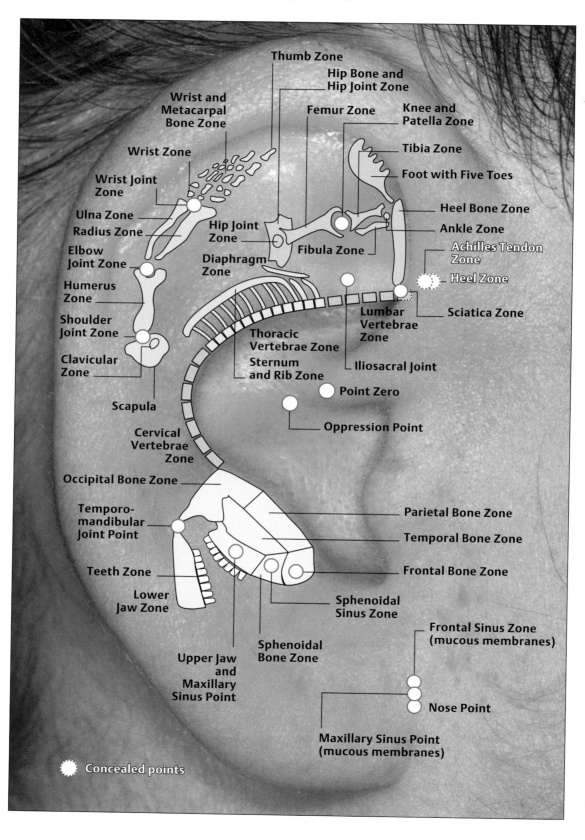

Topography of Important Projection Zones According to *Nogier*

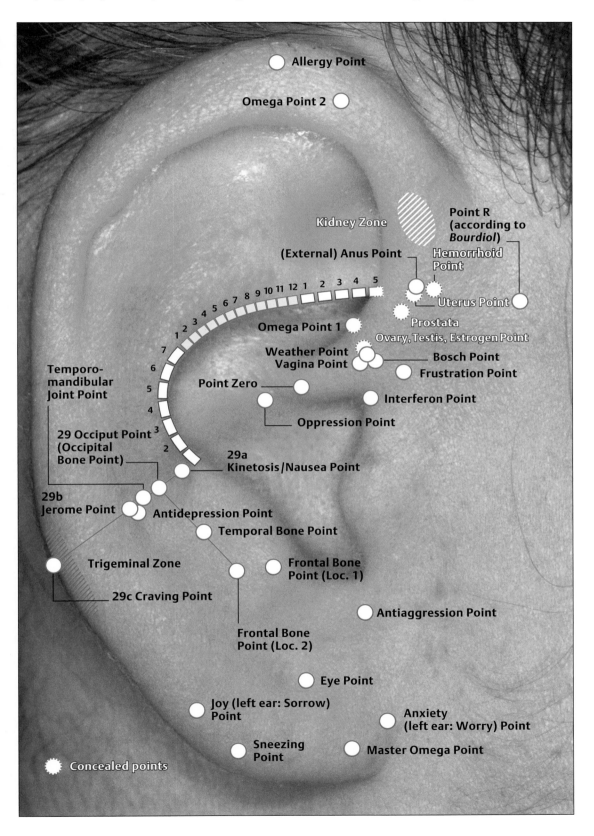

Allergy Point

Omega Point 2

Kidney Zone

Point R (according to *Bourdiol*)

(External) Anus Point

Hemorrhoid Point

Uterus Point

Omega Point 1

Prostata
Ovary, Testis, Estrogen Point

Weather Point
Vagina Point

Bosch Point

Frustration Point

Temporo-mandibular Joint Point

Point Zero

Interferon Point

Oppression Point

29 Occiput Point (Occipital Bone Point)

29a
Kinetosis/Nausea Point

29b Jerome Point

Antidepression Point

Temporal Bone Point

Trigeminal Zone

Frontal Bone Point (Loc. 1)

29c Craving Point

Antiaggression Point

Frontal Bone Point (Loc. 2)

Eye Point

Joy (left ear: Sorrow) Point

Anxiety (left ear: Worry) Point

Sneezing Point

Master Omega Point

Concealed points

Topography of Auricular Acupuncture Points
According to Chinese Nomenclature

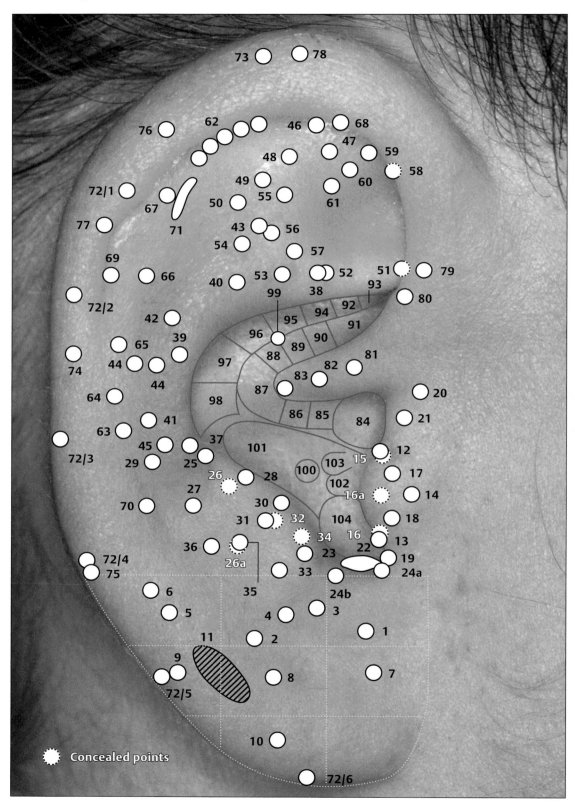

Auricular Acupuncture Points According to Chinese Nomenclature in Numerical Order and with Names

1 Analgesic Point for Tooth Extraction
2 Roof of Mouth Point
3 Floor of Mouth Point
4 Tongue Point
5 Upper Jaw Point
6 Lower Jaw Point
7 Analgesic Point for Toothache
8 Eye Point
9 Inner Ear Point
10 Tonsil Point
11 Cheek Zone
12 Apex of Tragus Point
13 Adrenal Gland Point
14 External Nose Point
15 Larynx, Pharynx Point
16 Inner Nose Point
16a Auriculotemporal Nerve
17 Thirst Point
18 Hunger Point
19 Hypertension Point
20 External Ear Point
21 Heart Point
22 Endocrine Zone
23 Ovary Point
24a Eye Point 1
24b Eye Point 2
25 Brain Stem Point
26 Toothache Point
26a Pituitary Gland Point
27 Larynx and Teeth Point
28 Brain Point
29 Epithelium Point
30 Parotid Gland Point
31 Asthma Point
32 Testis Point
33 Forehead Point
34 Gray Substance Point
35 Sun Point
36 Roof of Mouth Point
37 Cervical Vertebrae Point
38 Sacrum and Coccyx Vertebrae Point

39 Thoracic Vertebrae Zone (TVZ)
40 Lumbar Vertebrae Zone (LVZ)
41 Throat Point
42 Thorax Point
43 Abdomen Point
44 Mammary Gland Point
45 Thyroid Point
46 Toe Point
47 Heel Point
48 Ankle Point
49 Knee Joint Point
50 Hip Joint Zone
51 Vegetative System
52 Sciatic Nerve Zone
53 Posterior
54 Lumbar Vertebrae Pain Point
55 "Spirit Gate," *shen men*
56 Pelvis Point
57 Hip Point
58 Uterus Point
59 Blood Pressure–Reducing Point
60 Dyspnea Point
61 Hepatitis Point
62 Finger Point
63 Clavicula Point
64 Shoulder Joint Point
65 Shoulder Point
66 Elbow Point
67 Wrist Point
68 Appendix 1
69 Appendix 2
70 Appendix 3
71 Urticaria Zone
72 Helix (1–6)
73 Tonsil 1
74 Tonsil 2
75 Tonsil 3
76 Liver 1
77 Liver 2
78 Ear Tip Point

79 External Genitals Point
80 Urethra Point
81 Rectum Point
82 Diaphragm Point
83 Bifurcation Point
84 Mouth Zone
85 Esophagus Zone
86 Cardia Zone
87 Stomach Zone
88 Duodenum Zone
89 Small Intestine Zone
90 Appendix Zone 4
91 Colon Zone
92 Bladder Zone
93 Prostate Zone
94 Ureter Zone
95 Kidney Zone
96 Pancreas and Gallbladder Zone
97 Liver Zone
98 Spleen Zone
99 Ascites Point
100 Heart Zone
101 Lung Zone
102 Bronchial Zone
103 Trachea Zone
104 Triple Burner Zone
105 Blood Pressure–Reducing Furrow
106 Lower Back Point
107 Upper Back Point
108 Mid-Back Point

► Points 105–108 are located on the back of the ear.

Topography of Reflex Zones on the Auricula According to *R.A. Durinjan*

The Russian school has proposed another classification system of the auricula. In this system, a straight line is drawn from Point Zero through the Allergy Point (Point 78 "Tip of the Ear" according to Chinese nomenclature). Then additional straight lines are drawn at a distance of 30° from the helical rim so that the ear is finally divided by 12 straight lines that together form an angle of 360°. Within these zones the individual body sections are then projected.

Projection Zones of Head and Locomotor System

1–5	Fingers and Toes
6	Wrist
7	Forearm, Elbow Joint, and Upper Arm
8	Shoulder Joint, Thorax
9	Nape of the Neck Zone
10	Foot Zone
11	Lower Leg, Knee Joint
12	Thigh, Hip Joint
13	Lumbarsacral Zone
14	Upper Back and Stomach Zone
15	Lower Facial Zone and Larynx
16	Upper Facial Zone and Head with Associated Organs

Projection Zones of the Sexual System

I	Adenohypophysis
II	Main Erogenous Zone
III	Thalamic Zone
IV	Hypothalamic Zone
V	Zone of Lactation and Libido
VI	Zone of Libido and External Sexual Organs
VII	Zone of Suprarenal Glands
VIII	Antistress Zone
IX	Prostate, Ovary, and Uterus Zone
X	Libido Zone
XI	Zone of Sensory Influences on Sexual Functions
XII	Zone of Sensory Effects on Sexual Functions

Projection Zones of Internal Organs

1	Tactile and Gustatory Zone of the Lips, Tongue, and Oral Cavity
2	Pharynx and Esophagus
3	Stomach
4	Duodenum
5	Liver
6	Gallbladder
7	Pancreas
8	Kidneys
9	Bladder
10	Large Intestine
11	Diaphragm
12	Small Intestine
13	External Sexual Organs

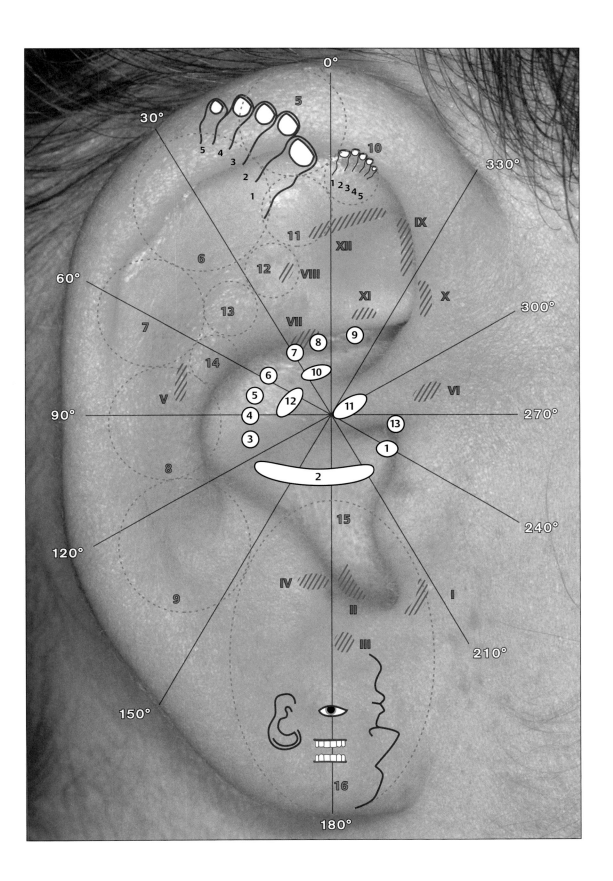

Projection Zones of the Sexual System According to *R.A. Durinjan*

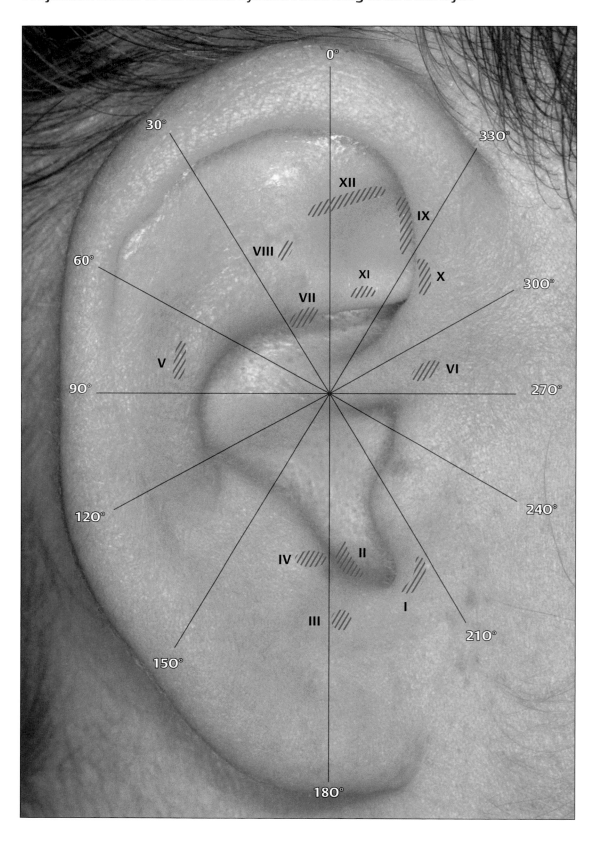

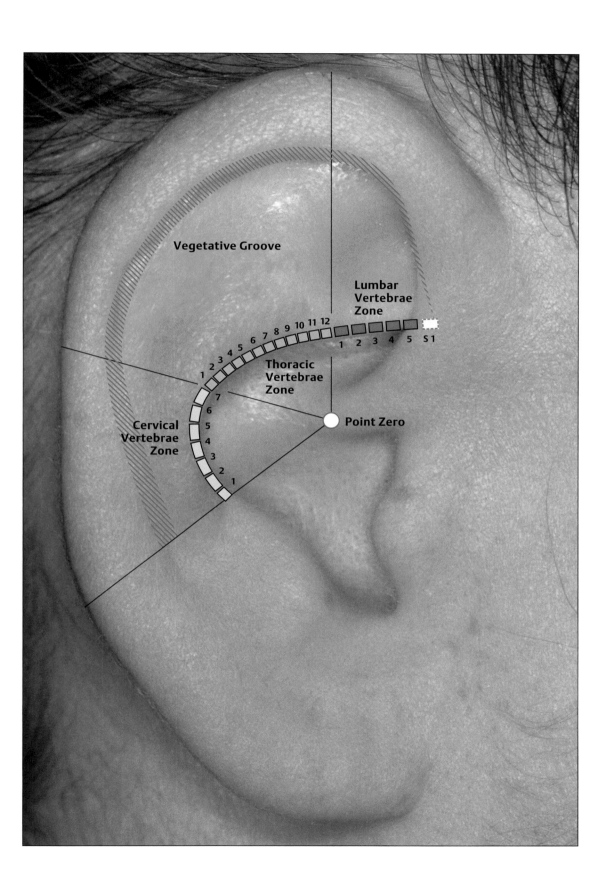

Vegetative Groove

Lumbar
Vertebrae
Zone

Thoracic
Vertebrae
Zone

Cervical
Vertebrae
Zone

Point Zero

Representation of the Ear Relief in Cross-Section and of Zones I–VIII According to *Nogier*

On account of the various curvatures in the anthe-lix from caudal to cranial, corresponding to cervi-cal, thoracic, and lumbar spinal column, cross sec-tions through the anthelix produce different relief forms. Various projection zones in the area of the scapha, anthelix, and concha can be distinguished.

The vertebrae are projected on the rim of the anthelix. The intervertebral disks follow the direc-tion of the concha. Further in the direction of the concha, the nerve control points of the endocrine glands are projected, the zone of the paravertebral sympathetic ganglia.

The zone of the organ parenchyma is projected in the concha itself.

We find the corresponding zones of the paraver-tebral muscles and ligaments in the area of the scapha. The spinal cord is projected on the rim with its motor, autonomic, and sensory tracts.

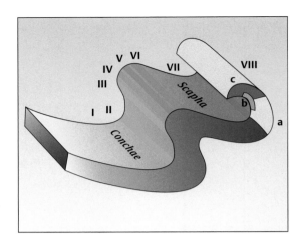

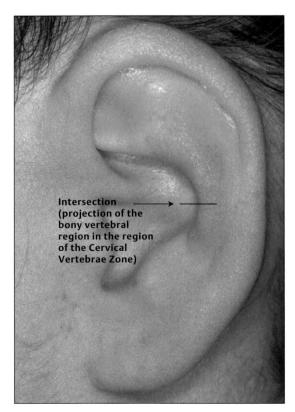

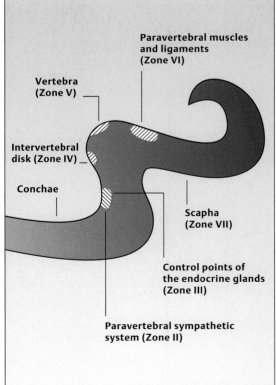

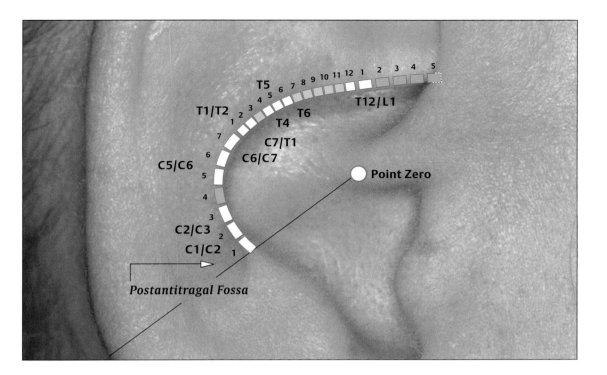

The Ear Relief in Cross-Section (Zones I–VIII)

I Zone of Organ Parenchyma

II Nervous Organ Points of the Paravertebral Chain of Sympathetic Ganglia

III Nervous Control Points of Endocrine Glands

IV Zone of Intervertebral Disks

V Vertebra Zone

VI Zone of Paravertebral Muscles and Ligaments

VII Vegetative Groove (Zone of Origin of Sympathetic Nuclei)

VIII Projection of the Spinal Cord
a: Motor tracts,
b: Autonomic tracts,
c: Sensory tracts.

Nervous Control Points of Endocrine Glands

T12/L1	Zone III, Suprarenal Gland Point*
T6	Zone III, Suprarenal Gland Point*
T12	Zone III, Pancreas Point*
T6	Zone III, Pancreas Point*
T4	Zone III, Thymus Gland Point*
T1/T2	Zone III, Thymus Gland Point*
T5	Zone III, Mammary Gland Point
C6/C7	Zone III, Thyroid Gland Point
C5/C6	Zone III, Parathyroid Gland Point

* Depending on affiliation with one or the other school, the localization of different points may vary.

Nervous Organ Points of the Paravertebral Chain of Sympathetic Ganglia

C1/C2	Zone II, Superior Cervical Ganglion Point
C2/C3	Zone II, Middle Cervical Ganglion Point
C7/T1	Zone II, Inferior Cervical Ganglion Point (Stellate Ganglion Point)

Significance of Laterality

When examining the reflex zones in the ear, as a rule we will find different reactive points in the right and left ear. In principle, regardless of laterality, in auricular acupuncture we only find active auricular acupuncture points if there is a corresponding disturbance in the corresponding part of the body or functional relationship. In a healthy, balanced patient at best no auricular acupuncture point can be actively demonstrated. Besides being of therapeutic value, this is also of diagnostic relevance.

NOTE *Orthodox medical diagnosis takes absolute priority. Diagnosis via the auricula or another somatope can provide valuable additional information.*

Most patients are right-handed with a dominant left cerebral hemisphere. As a rule, here we find increased reactivity in the area of the right ear. In those who are left-handed, we often find increased reactivity in the area of the left ear.

In general, it may be said that disturbances with an organpathological basis may be treated via the ear on the side on which the organpathological alteration is found. Thus, for example, pain in the region of the right knee joint is generally treated via the right ear, pain in the region of the left knee joint via the left ear. This means that, regardless of whether the patient is left or right-handed, the disturbance is treated homolaterally depending on the organpathological localization.

This also applies to the internal organs. Pain in the region of the right kidney, for example, is treated via the right ear, pain in the region of the left kidney via the left ear.

The laterality of organs located in the middle, i.e., bladder, prostate, uterus, and trachea, is more difficult to establish. As a rule, treatment of those who are right-handed is via the right ear and those who are left-handed via the left ear. The rule which may be applied is that treatment is principally conducted via the "ear calling out for treatment," in other words, the ear in which the most responsive points are found.

It is often very difficult to establish precise laterality. In such cases, treatment via both ears is recommended.

Nogier's Reflex (ACR) is an important tool in determining laterality for the acupuncturist trained and experienced in auricular medicine (cf. p. 30).

It should be pointed out that the problem of laterality is a very controversial topic for the different schools.

The only criterion for the right approach is the success of the therapy. Successes and failures, regardless of affiliation with one or the other school, mark the path of every experienced acupuncturist.

Laterality Disturbances

In laterality disturbances we find an unclear assignment of active auricular acupuncture points in both ears. Unequivocal dominance cannot be demonstrated on the basis of the findings. Accordingly, therefore, we do not find active auricular acupuncture points in the dominant ear, but active auricular acupuncture points in both ears.

In such cases, the laterality control point is frequently needled therapeutically. This is roughly 3 cm from the middle of the tragus in the direction of the face.

Hyperresponsiveness or hyporesponsiveness is frequently found in combination with laterality disturbances in the ear. In hyperresponsiveness, almost every point represents an active point; in hyporesponsiveness it is possible for no active points at all to be found.

In such cases, needling with silver or gold needles has proved worthwhile: In hyperresponsiveness, needling of Point Zero is performed with a silver needle, in hyporesponsiveness with a gold needle.

Simple methods for ascertaining laterality are well known, thus, for example

- ► The dominant hand is on top when clapping.

- ► Which hand is used to perform difficult tasks?

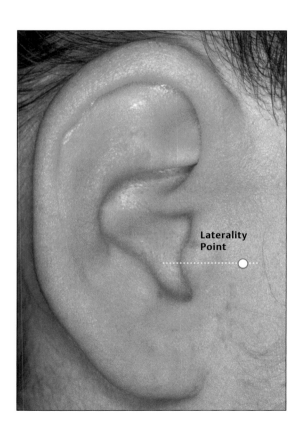

Laterality Point

Rule for the Selection of Auricular Acupuncture Points

Nogier School, Auricular Geometry According to *Nogier*

According to *Nogier,* we often find important pain and treatment points in the region of the ear which are all located in a line. Starting from Point Zero, the irritated vertebra is sought. From Point Zero a straight line is drawn through this point (irritated vertebra) to the Vegetative Groove. The end of this line is in the Vegetative Groove. From this line a second support line is drawn at an angle of 30° or a multiple angle of 30° (60°, 90°). The interfaces of this support line with the Vegetative Groove and the helix represent important additional control points.

Nogier and *Bourdiol* call the Vegetative Groove the "zone of neurovegetative medullar centers." Today, however, we know that the projection of the medullar centers only covers a much smaller region. Nonetheless, these are, of course, energetically effective points.

Nogier's Reflex
Auriculocardiac Reflex (ACR)
Vascular Autonomic Signal (VAS)

Underlying *Nogier's* Reflex is a cutaneovascular reflex discovered by *Nogier* in 1968. He noticed a change in the pulse wave of the radial artery when irritated ear points or zones are stimulated. While doing so, he observed two phenomena: an increase in pulse strength, which he called positive ACR, and a decrease in pulse strength, which he called negative ACR. Today we know that in both cases the same sympathetic reflex response is involved and that a positively or negatively experienced pulse reflex only depends on the position of the thumb taking the pulse. We therefore now only speak of the ACR or *Nogier's* Reflex (known as the Vascular Autonomic Signal [VAS] internationally).

For the *Nogier* school, this is the most important approach when selecting acupuncture points. The school of auriculomedicine differs significantly from the Chinese school in this respect.

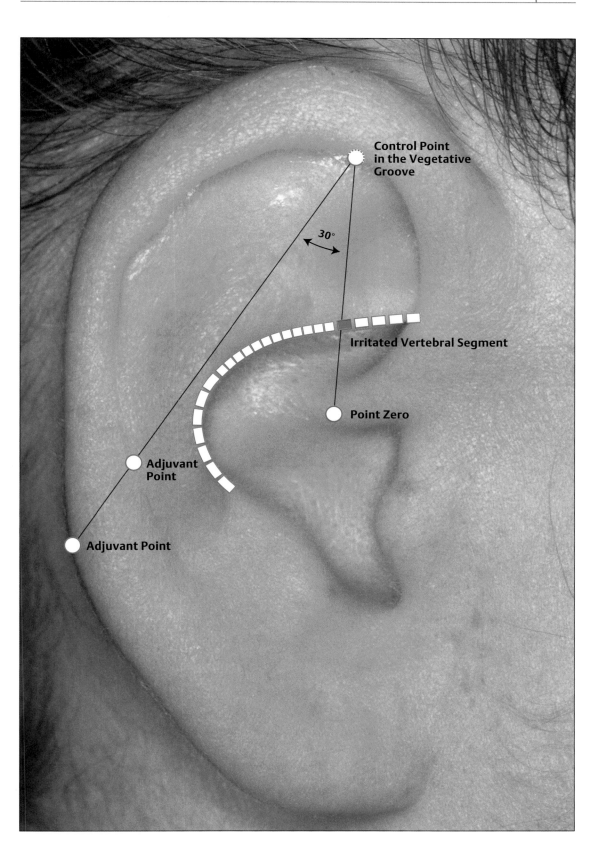

Control Point
in the Vegetative
Groove

30°

Irritated Vertebral Segment

Point Zero

Adjuvant
Point

Adjuvant Point

Chinese School

In accordance with the various schools of auricular acupuncture, there are various approaches to the selection of acupuncture points for needling. Selection is frequently made according to their "importance" or corresponding zones. Thus, in the case of stomach complaints the Stomach Point of auricular acupuncture is needled, in the case of complaints of the vertebral column the corresponding acupuncture point of the vertebral column.

Every treatment is preceded by an examination of the patient and the ear. In the region of the auricula, we frequently find places which are painful when pressure is applied (trigger points). These can also give us diagnostic information. According to the findings of the examination, these particularly conspicuous points are included in the treatment program.

Another option for point selection presupposes a knowledge and understanding of Traditional Chinese Medicine (TCM). Here the points may be selected according to the relationships represented in TCM. In skin diseases, for example, the Lung Point is needled, as the skin is connected to the lung in accordance with the Theory of the Five Elements.

According to the coupling relationships of TCM (*yin–yang* coupling, top-to-bottom coupling), there are additional options for point selection.

The auricular acupuncture points can therefore be selected according to various criteria.

1. According to Structural Considerations

Irritations, for example, in the region of the CVZ

▶ Needling of the corresponding acupuncture point of the CVZ

2. According to Functional Considerations

Here the rules of TCM are applied, for example:

Headache at the back of the head

▶ Treatment via the *tai yang* axis, Small Intestine—Bladder

Sleep disturbances, palpitations

▶ Heart Point

3. According to Pathophysiological Considerations

Dysmenorrhea

▶ Endocrine Point, Pituitary Gland Point

Hypertonus

▶ Blood Pressure–Reducing Furrow Zone

4. According to Clinical Experience

Inflammatory eye diseases

▶ Eye Point

4 Tongue Point

Location: Quadrant II, center.

Indication: Stomatitis, toothache.

5 Upper Jaw Point

Location: Quadrant III, roughly in the middle.

Indication: Trigeminal neuralgia.

6 Lower Jaw Point

Location: Quadrant III, upper demarcation of the field.

Indication: Trigeminal neuralgia, toothache.

7 Analgesic Point for Tooth Extraction

Location: Quadrant IV, center.

Indication: Tooth extraction, migraine.

8 Eye Point ⊙

Location: Quadrant V, center.

Indication: Inflammatory eye disorders, hordeolum, glaucoma, cephalalgia that radiates into the eyes.

9 Inner Ear Point ⊙

Location: Quadrant VI, in the middle.

Indication: Vertigo, tinnitus, impaired hearing.

10 Tonsil Point

Location: Quadrant VIII, center.

Indication: The point has lymphatic activity.

11 Cheek Zone

Location: Quadrants V and VI.

Indication: Facial paresis, trigeminal neuralgia.

For comparison: Points on the lobule according to Nogier

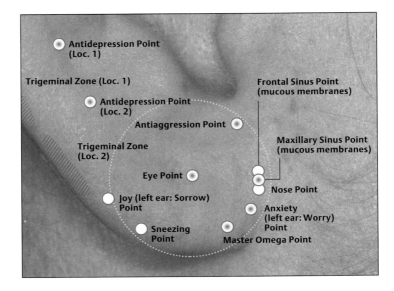

Points on the Lobule According to *Nogier*

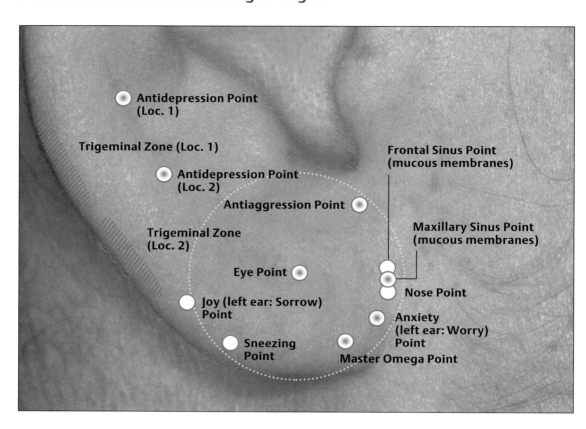

Trigeminal Zone

(Different locations are indicated, depending on affiliation with one or the other school.)

Location 1: On the lateral, upper edge of the lobule

Location 2: In a more caudal location, dorsal demarcation of the fields (cf. Chinese points 6 [Lower Jaw Point] and 9 [Inner Ear Point]).

Indication: Trigeminal neuralgia.

> ► Pricking technique: Use the needle to prick the area of the trigeminal zone and possibly let it bleed. Prick electrically active or pressure-sensitive point with gold needle.

Eye Point ◉

Location: In the middle of the lobule.

Indication: Eye disorders, migraine, pollinosis.

Sneezing Point

Location: On the lower lateral part of the lobule.

Indication: Pollinosis.

Antiaggression Point ◉

Location: At the lower edge of the intertragic notch, toward the face.

Indication: An important psychotropic point; addiction treatment (a silver point on the dominant ear).

Master Omega Point ◉

Location: On the caudal part of the lobule toward the face.

Indication: An important psychotropic point; intensely effective, harmonizes the vegetative system.

Antidepression Point ⊚

(Different locations are indicated, depending on affiliation with one or the other school.)

Location 1: On the elongation of the Vegetative Groove, on a line which runs through Point Zero and C1.

Location 2: On the nasocaudal side of the Jerome Point, on the cranial side of the intersection of the Vegetative Groove with a straight line through the Antiaggression Point.

Indication: Depressive mood, psychosomatic disturbances.

Anxiety/Worry Point ⊚

Location: On the front edge of the lobule at the point where it emerges, at eye level.

Indication: Anxiety, worry. In case of right-handedness:

- ► Anxiety: Treatment via the right ear (silver needle);
- ► Worry: Treatment via the left ear (silver needle).

In case of left-handedness: vice versa.

Nose Point

Location: Just below the Maxillary Sinus Zone.

Indication: Rhinitis, pollinosis.

Point of Sorrow and Joy

Location: On the occipital part of the lobule, at the same level as the Anxiety Zone.

Indication: Sorrow, joy.

- ► Impaired zest for life: Treatment via the right ear,
- ► Sorrow: Treatment via the left ear.

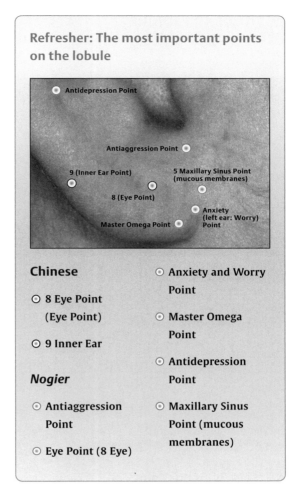

Refresher: The most important points on the lobule

- Antidepression Point
- Antiaggression Point
- 9 (Inner Ear Point)
- 5 Maxillary Sinus Point (mucous membranes)
- 8 (Eye Point)
- Anxiety (left ear: Worry) Point
- Master Omega Point

Chinese

- ⊙ 8 Eye Point (Eye Point)
- ⊙ 9 Inner Ear

Nogier

- ⊙ Antiaggression Point
- ⊙ Eye Point (8 Eye)

- ⊙ Anxiety and Worry Point
- ⊙ Master Omega Point
- ⊙ Antidepression Point
- ⊙ Maxillary Sinus Point (mucous membranes)

Maxillary Sinus Point ⊚ (Mucous Membranes)

Location: In the middle of the point where the lobule emerges in the skin of the face.

Indication: Afflictions of the nasal sinuses, field of disturbance.

Frontal Sinus Point (Mucous Membranes)

Location: On the cranial side of the Frontal Sinus Zone.

Indication: Afflictions of the nasal sinuses, field of disturbance.

Points on the Tragus (12–19) and Supratragic Notch (20 and 21) According to Chinese Nomenclature

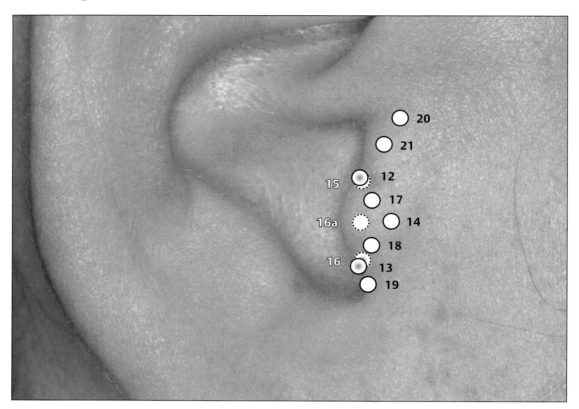

12 Apex of Tragus Point ⊙

Location: On the cranial side of a single-peaked tragus. On the cranial peak of a double-peaked tragus.

Indication: Analgesia. The point has anti-inflammatory activity.

13 Adrenal Gland Point ⊙

Location: On the lower third of a single-peaked tragus. On the caudal peak of a double-peaked tragus.

Indication: Allergic diathesis, joint disorders, chronic inflammation, functional circulatory disorders, paresis, neuralgia. Generally indicated in all forms of adrenal gland dysfunction.

14 External Nose Point

Location: In the middle of the base of the tragus.

Indication: Local afflictions of the nose (eczema, rhinophyma, etc.).

15 Larynx, Pharynx Point

Location: On the inside of the tragus at the level of Point 12.

Indication: Pharyngitis, tonsillitis.

▶ Caution: Caution: Danger of collapse (vagus irritation).

16 Inner Nose Point ⊙

Location: On the inside of the tragus at the level of Point 13.

Indication: Rhinitis, sinusitis.

▶ Caution: Danger of collapse (vagus irritation).

16a Auriculotemporal Nerve

Location: Between Point 15 and Point 16, inside.

Indication: Neuralgia in the innervation zone of the nerve.

17 Thirst Point

Location: Midway between Point 12 and Point 14.

Indication: Thirst, bulimia.

18 Hunger Point

Location: Midway between Point 13 and Point 14.

Indication: For example, weight reduction.

19 Hypertension Point

Location: At the transition to the intertragic notch.

▶ According to *Nogier,* the ACTH Point is at this location.

Indication: Hypertension.

20 External Ear Point

Location: Roughly corresponds to TB-21 in body acupuncture.

Indication: Inflammation of the external ear, tinnitus, hearing difficulties.

21 Heart Point

Location: Roughly in the middle of the connecting line between Point 20 and Point 12.

Indication: Functional heart complaints.

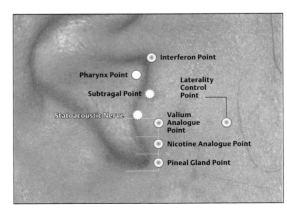

For comparison: Points on the tragus and supratragic notch according to Nogier *and* Bahr

Points on the Tragus and Supratragic Notch According to *Nogier*

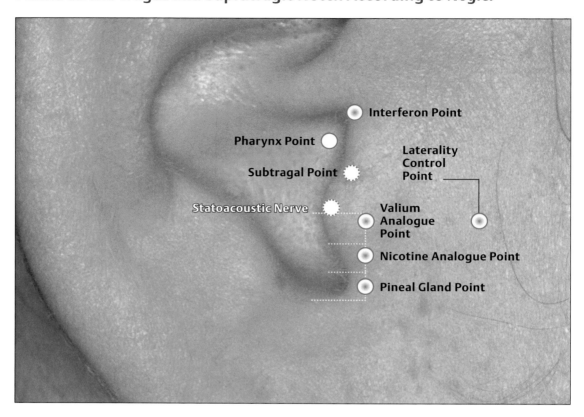

How to Find the Points

A horizontal line through the middle of the tragus and another line through the bottom of the inter-tragic notch are connected by a vertical line roughly 3 mm in front of the tragus edge. The distance between the two lines is divided into thirds. In the middle of each subsection is located one of the following points: Valium Analogue Point, Nicotine Analogue Point, and Pineal Gland Point.

Larynx/Pharynx Point

Location: At the top end of the tragus, in the cavity of concha.

Indication: Afflictions in the neck area, globus sensation, addiction treatment.

Interferon Point

Location: In the supratragic notch (gold point on the non-dominant ear).

Indication: The point has an immuno-modulating effect and anti-inflammatory activity.

Valium Analogue Point

Location: On the tragus, roughly 2 mm before the edge of the tragus and just below the middle of the tragus (gold point on non-dominant ear).

Indication: Addiction treatment; the point has general sedating activity.

Nicotine Analogue Point

Location: Just below the Valium Analogue Point (gold point on the non-dominant ear).

Indication: Addiction treatment.

Pineal Gland Point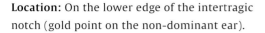

Location: On the lower edge of the intertragic notch (gold point on the non-dominant ear).

Indication: Disturbed circadian rhythm; an adjuvant point in hormonal disorders.

Subtragal Point

Location: On the inside of the tragus, cranial side.

Indication: Control point of reticular formation, overall vegetative harmonization, antioscillatory. (Normally an identical stimulus provoked in the body will involve the same reflex response every time. For example, the response to the point-searching device will always be identical or the number of pulse beats will always be the same while the pressure of the pressure button on the skin is the same. On the other hand, if the patient is oscillating, the body will respond to an identical stimulus in different ways every time, i.e. an auricular point will be found on one occasion and then not on another—the reflex response of the organism is unstable. Disturbed routing of stimuli in reticular formation is assumed to be the cause.)

Laterality Control Point *(Bahr)* ⊙

Location: On a horizontal line roughly 3 cm from the middle of the tragus.

Indication: Laterality disturbances (gold point on the dominant ear).

Statoacoustic Nerve

Location: Tip of the tragus.

Indication: Ménière disease, vertigo.

► Possible needling in combination with the Stellate Ganglion Zone.

Refresher: The most important points on the tragus and supratragic notch

- Interferon Point
- Laterality Control Point
- 12 12
- Valium Analogue Point
- 16 13
- Nicotine Analogue Point
- Pineal Gland Point

Chinese	Nogier/Bahr
⊙ 12 Apex of Tragus Point	⊙ Valium Analogue Point
⊙ 13 Adrenal Gland Point	⊙ Nicotine Analogue Point
⊙ 16 Inner Nose Point	⊙ Pineal Gland Point
	⊙ Laterality Point
	⊙ Interferon Point

For comparison: Points 12–21 on the tragus and supratragic notch according to Chinese nomenclature

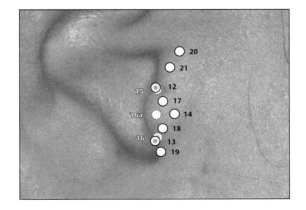

Points on the Intertragic Notch (Points 22–24) According to Chinese Nomenclature

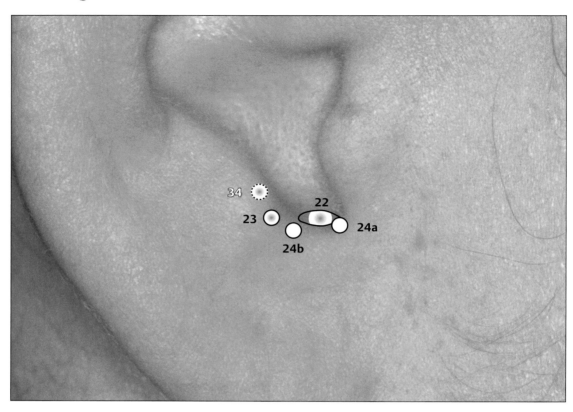

22 Endocrine Zone ⊙

Location: At the bottom of the intertragic notch, toward the face.

Indication: All endocrine disorders (gynecological and rheumatoid disorders, allergies, skin disorders).

▸ According to *Nogier*, this zone corresponds to the points of the adrenal gland, thyroid gland, and parathyroid gland.

23 Ovary Point ⊙ (Gonadotropin Point According to *Nogier*)

Location: On the ventral and outer ridge of the antitragus, "Eye of the Snake," when viewing anthelix as a snake.

Indication: Ovarian dysfunction, menstruation-related migraines, skin disorders.

24a Eye Point 1

Location: Below the intertragic notch, toward the face.

Indication: Non-inflammatory eye disorders, possibly myopia, astigmatism, opticus atrophy.

24b Eye Point 2

Location: Below the intertragic notch, in the direction of the helix.

Indication: Non-inflammatory eye disorders, possibly myopia, astigmatism, opticus atrophy.

28 Brain Point (Pituitary Gland Point)

Location: In the middle of the line from the peak of the antitragus to the anthelix–antitragus intersection.

Indication: Hormone dysfunction.

29 Occiput Point ⊙ (Occipital Bone Point According to *Nogier*)

Location: Roughly midway between the Vegetative Groove and Point 25, Brain Stem, in the postantitragal fossa.

Indication: Broad spectrum of activity: conditions of pain, autonomic dysfunction, recovery phases.

30 Parotid Gland Point ⊙

Location: On the tip of the antitragus.

Indication: Pruritus (strong antipruritic effect), inflammation of the parotid gland, mumps.

31 Asthma Point ⊙

Location: Below the tip of the antitragus in the direction of the base of the antitragus.

Indication: Bronchitis, asthma. The point affects the respiratory center.

32 Testis Point

Location: On the inside of the antitragus, corresponding to the external location of Point 31.

Indication: Impotence, orchitis.

33 Forehead Point ⊙ (Frontal Bone Point According to *Nogier*)

Location: End point of the Sensory Line (*Nogier* calls the line connecting Points 29, 35, and 33 the Sensory Line), roughly at the level of a horizontal line through the middle of the caudal tragus side.

Indication: Disturbances (-algia, -itis) in the forehead region, vertigo.

34 Gray Substance Point ⊙ (Vegetative Point II According to *Nogier*)

Location: On the inside of the antitragus, above the Ovary Point (23).

Indication: The point has a general harmonizing effect, antiphlogistic activity and analgesic activity.

35 Sun Point ⊙ (Temporal Bone Point According to *Nogier*)

Location: In the middle of the base of the antitragus.

Indication: Very frequently used point. Cephalgia, migraine, eye disorders, vertigo, insomnia.

36 Roof of Mouth Point

Location: Below Point 29.

Indication: Frontal headache.

For comparison:
Points on the antitragus
according to Nogier

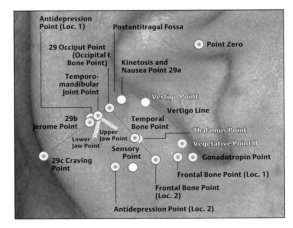

Points on the Antitragus According to *Nogier*

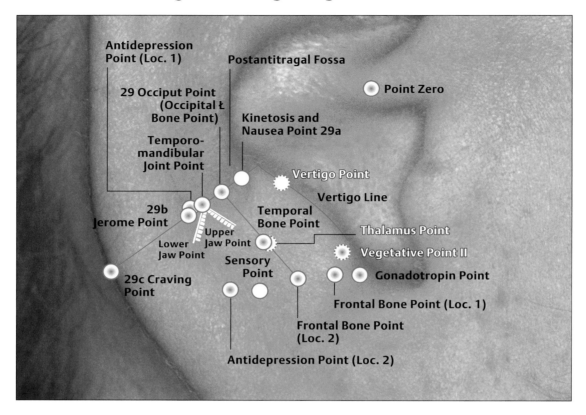

Postantitragal Fossa

Location: A straight line is drawn from Point Zero through the notch between the antitragus and anthelix to the edge of the ear. Important acupuncture points (29a, 29, 29b, 29c) are located on this line. We call the line connecting them the postantitragal fossa.

Indication: For details, see the respective points.

Sensory Line

Nogier calls the line between the Frontal Bone Point (33, Forehead Point), Temporal Bone Point (35, Sun Point), and Occipital Bone Point (29, Occiput Point) the Sensory Line. Energetic blood flow to the head is assigned to this line, as is the case with the body acupuncture points Ex-HN-3 and GV-16 (*Bischko*).

The postantitragal fossa and the Sensory Line represent two basic pillars of ear acupuncture treatment. The respective conspicuous points may be used together with the related spinal column segment for basic therapy in pain treatment.

Occipital Bone Point, Occiput Point ⊙ (29   Occiput Point According to Chinese Nomenclature)

Location: In the postantitragal fossa, roughly midway between Point 29a and Point 29b. According to Chinese nomenclature, the localization of the Occiput Point is slightly more toward the face.

Indication: An important analgesic point with a broad spectrum of activity. Conditions of pain, vertigo, autonomic dysfunction, phase of recovery.

29a Kinetosis and Nausea Point

Location: Between the anthelical edge and Point 29 (Occiput Point).

Indication: Kinetosis, vomiting.

29b Jerome Point
Relaxation Point

Location: In the postantitragal fossa, at the intersection with the Vegetative Groove.

Indication: For vegetative harmonization. Difficulty falling asleep. In case of difficulty staying asleep, the corresponding point on the back of the ear is needled. This relaxes the muscles.

29c Craving Point

Location: At the end of the postantitragal fossa, at the intersection with the edge of the ear.

Indication: Used within the scope of addiction therapy.

Vertigo Point

Location: On the inside in the area of the antitragus, shortly before the postantitragal fossa.

Indication: Important vertigo point, cf. Vertigo Line according to *von Steinburg*.

Temporomandibular Joint Point

Location: The point is at the end of the scapha, at the transition to the ear lobe.
In the area of the temporomandibular joint we also find the projection zones

- a) Palatine tonsil
- b) Molars of the upper and lower jaw
- c) Retromolar area
- d) Rear sections of the masticatory muscles
- e) Antidepression Point (cf. p. 41 and 55)
- f) Magnesium Point (*Bahr*)
- g) Parotid Gland Point
- h) Base of the lateral pterygoid muscle.

Indication: Gnathological problems, pain syndrome, tinnitus.

Frontal Bone Point
(33 Forehead Point
According to Chinese Nomenclature)

(Depending on the affiliation with one or the other school, different locations are indicated.)

Location 1: On the ventral part of the antitragus, almost at the intersection with the intertragic notch.

Location 2: End point of the Sensory Line (*Nogier* calls the line connecting Points 29, 35 and 33 the Sensory Line), roughly at the level of a horizontal line through the middle of the caudal tragus side.

Indication: Disturbances (-algia, -itis) in the forehead region, vertigo.

Temporal Bone Point
(35 Sun Point
According to Chinese Nomenclature)

Location: In the middle of the base of the antitragus.

Indication: Cephalgia, vertigo, conditions of pain.

Upper Jaw Point (incl. Teeth)

Location: Starting from the temporomandibular joint on the mediocaudal side.

Indication: Pain and disturbances in the region of the upper jaw/teeth.

Lower Jaw Point (incl. Teeth)

Location: Starting from the temporomandibular joint on the caudal, lateral side.

Indication: Pain and disturbances in the region of the lower jaw/teeth.

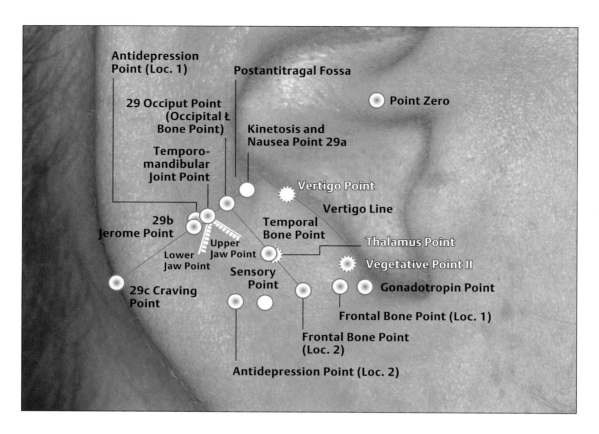

Sensory Point

Location: On the caudal side of the Temporal Bone Point (35, Sun Point according to Chinese nomenclature).

Indication: Pain relief.

Vegetative System II

(34 Gray Substance Point According to Chinese Nomenclature)

Location: On the inside of the antitragus, on the caudal leg.

Indication: Analgesic, vegetative harmonization.

Vertigo Line According to *von Steinburg*

Location: Along the postantitragal fossa and upper edge of the antitragus, slightly on the inside.

Indication: Vertigo.

Gonadotropin Point

Location: On the ventral and outer edge of the antitragus ("Eye of the Snake," when viewing the anthelix as a snake).

Indication: Sexual dysfunction, dysmenorrhea, amenorrhea.

Vertigo Line according to von Steinburg

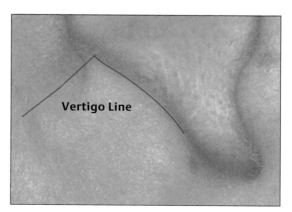

Thalamus Point
(26a Pituitary Gland Point According to Chinese Nomenclature)

Location: On the inside of the antitragus, opposite the Temporal Bone Point (Point 35, Sun Point, according to Chinese nomenclature).

Indication: Vegetative harmonization, a general analgesic point, premature ejaculation, frigidity; affects the homolateral side of the body.

▶ In case of articular rheumatism: use gold needles.

▶ Caution: Contraindicated during pregnancy.

Antidepression Point ⊙
(Different locations are indicated, depending on affiliation with one or the other school.)

Location 1: On the elongation of the Vegetative Groove, on a line which runs through Point Zero and C1.

Location 2: On the nasocaudal side of the Jerome Point, on the cranial side of the intersection of the Vegetative Groove with a straight line through the Antiaggression Point.

Indication: Depressive mood, psychosomatic disturbances.

For comparison:
Points on the antitragus
according to Chinese nomenclature

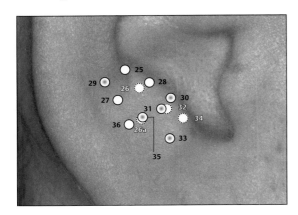

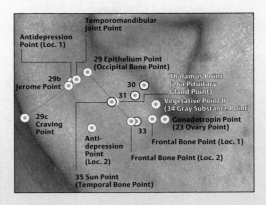

Refresher: The most important points on the antitragus

Chinese	Nogier
⊙ 23 Ovary Point (Gonadotropin Point)	⊙ 29 Epithelium Point (Occipital Bone Point)
⊙ 26a Pituitary Gland Point (Thalamus Point)	⊙ 29b Jerome Point
	⊙ 29c Craving Point
⊙ 29 Epithelium Point (Occipital Bone Point)	⊛ Vegetative Point II (34 Gray Substance Point)
⊙ 30 Parotid Gland Point	⊛ Thalamus Point (26a Pituitary Gland Point)
⊙ 31 Asthma Point	⊙ Gonadotropin Point (23 Ovary Point)
⊙ 33 Forehead Point (Frontal Bone Point)	⊙ Temporomandibular Joint Point
⊛ 34 Gray Substance Point (Vegetative Point II)	⊙ Antidepression Point
⊙ 35 Sun Point (Temporal Bone Point)	⊙ Frontal Bone Point (33 Forehead Point)
	⊙ Temporal Bone Point (35 Sun Point)

Projection Zones of the Cranial Bones and Sinuses According to *Nogier*

The cranial bones are projected on the area of the antitragus. The frontal bone is represented on the ascending part of the antitragus. The ethmoid bone and the upper jaw are projected more toward the helical rim. The parietal bone is represented in the ventral area on the apex of the antitragus. The projection of the occipital bone forms the border in a dorsal direction. The temporal bone is projected in the middle of the antitragus. The temporomandibular joint and the lower jaw with the teeth join the occipital bone.

As a field of disturbance, the paranasal sinuses play a major role. They are also projected in the antitragus region (bony part of the maxillary sinuses, at the height of the upper jaw). However, the mucus membrane part of the maxillary sinuses is in the area in which the nose is located at the front edge of the ear lobe. The frontal sinus is slightly below the frontal bone. The sphenoidal and ethmoidal sinuses are projected on a line in the immediate vicinity of the maxillary sinus.

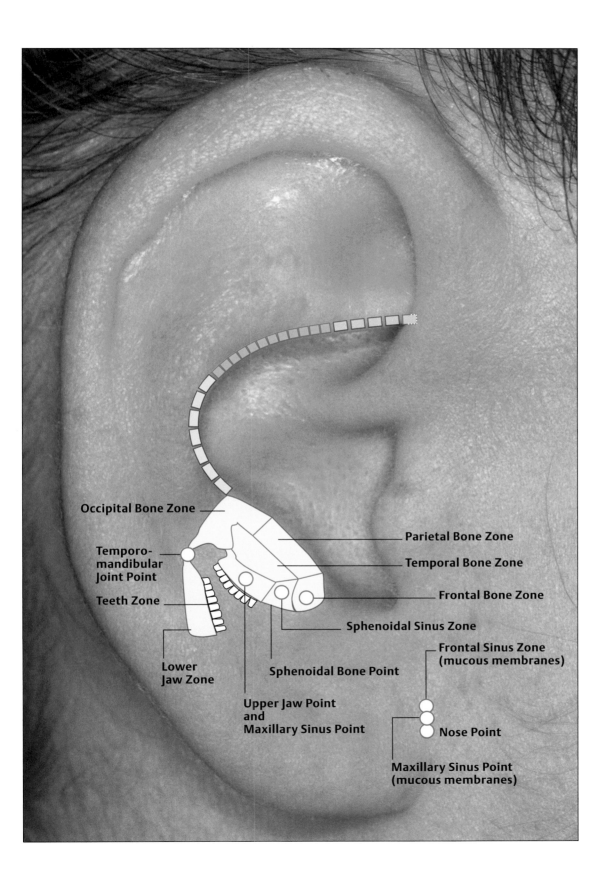

Occipital Bone Zone

Temporo-
mandibular
Joint Point

Teeth Zone

Lower
Jaw Zone

Parietal Bone Zone

Temporal Bone Zone

Frontal Bone Zone

Sphenoidal Sinus Zone

Sphenoidal Bone Point

Upper Jaw Point
and
Maxillary Sinus Point

Frontal Sinus Zone
(mucous membranes)

Nose Point

Maxillary Sinus Point
(mucous membranes)

Topography and Indications

Points of the Anthelix (Points 37–45) According to Chinese Nomenclature

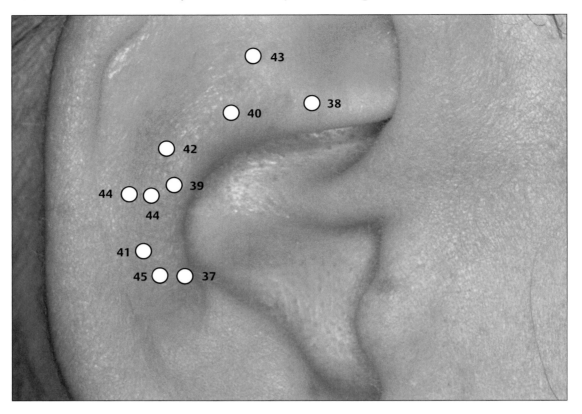

Unlike the differentiated representation of the spinal column in the area of the anthelix according to *Nogier*, Chinese auricular acupuncture in part only indicates individual points for the corresponding vertebral segments. These might correspond to maximum points. The responsiveness of the corresponding auricular acupuncture point is decisive.

37   Cervical Vertebrae Point

Location: In the caudal area of the antitragus.

Indication: Cervical vertebrae syndrome.

38   Sacrum and Coccyx Vertebrae Point

Location: At the level of the intersection at the crura, on the anthelix.

Indication: Lumbar vertebrae syndrome, coxalgia.

39   Thoracic Vertebrae Zone

Location: In the elongation of the ascending root of helix to the helix, on the anthelix.

Indication: Thoracodynia, pain in the thorax.

50 Hip Point ⊙

Location: On the caudal side of the projection zone for the knee joint, above the point at which both anthelical crura meet on the superior anthelical crus.

Indication: Pain in the hip region.

51 Vegetative Point ☺

Location: At the intersection of the inferior anthelical crus and the helix.

Indication: An important point; vegetative stabilization of all visceral organs.

52 Sciatic Nerve Point ⊙

Location: Roughly in the center of the inferior anthelical crus.

Indication: Pain in the innervation area of the sciatic nerve.

53 Posterior Point

Location: Lateral to Point 52.

Indication: Pain in the posterior region.

54 Loin Pain Point

Location: At the intersection of the superior and inferior anthelical crura.

Indication: Pain in the loin region.

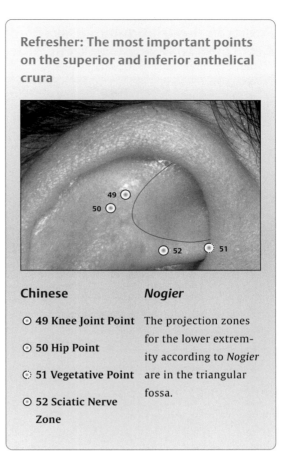

Refresher: The most important points on the superior and inferior anthelical crura

Chinese	Nogier
⊙ 49 Knee Joint Point	The projection zones for the lower extremity according to *Nogier* are in the triangular fossa.
⊙ 50 Hip Point	
☺ 51 Vegetative Point	
⊙ 52 Sciatic Nerve Zone	

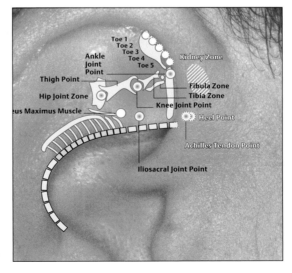

*For comparison:
Points on the superior and
inferior anthelical crura
and the triangular fossa
according to* Nogier

Points in the Triangular Fossa (Points 55–61)
According to Chinese Nomenclature

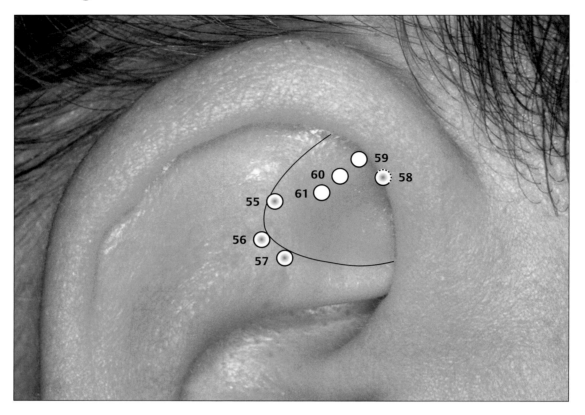

55 *Shen men* (Spirit Gate) ◉

Location: In the angle formed by the superior and inferior anthelical crura, more toward the superior anthelical crus.

Indication: An important point. Very effective for emotional stabilization; a point of overriding importance in conditions of pain, anti-inflammatory activity; frequently used as part of the treatment of *yang* diseases.

56 Pelvis Point ◉

Location: In the angle formed by the superior and inferior anthelical crura.

Indication: Pain in the pelvic area.

▶ Hip Point and Pelvis Point according to *Nogier* are identical with Point 56.

57 Hip Point ◉

Location: On the inside the inferior anthelical crus, on the caudal side of the intersection area of both anthelical crura.

Indication: Pain in the hip region.

58 Uterus Point ◉

Location: In the triangular fossa, cranial portion, partially below the helix.

Indication: Condition after uterus extirpation, for example, postoperative pain.

59 Blood Pressure–Reduction Point

Location: At the intersection of the superior anthelical crus and helix in the direction of the triangular fossa.

Indication: Hypertension, possibly microphlebotomy.

60 Dyspnea Point

Location: Caudal and lateral to Point 59 on a level with the Uterus Point (58).

Indication: Bronchial asthma.

61 Hepatitis Point

Location: Lateral to Point 58 on the edge of the superior anthelical crus.

Indication: Adjuvant point in liver diseases.

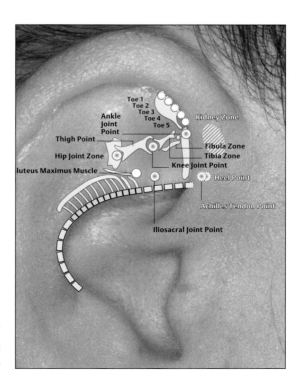

For comparison:
Points on the triangular fossa
according to Nogier

Projection Zones of the Lower Extremity According to *Nogier*

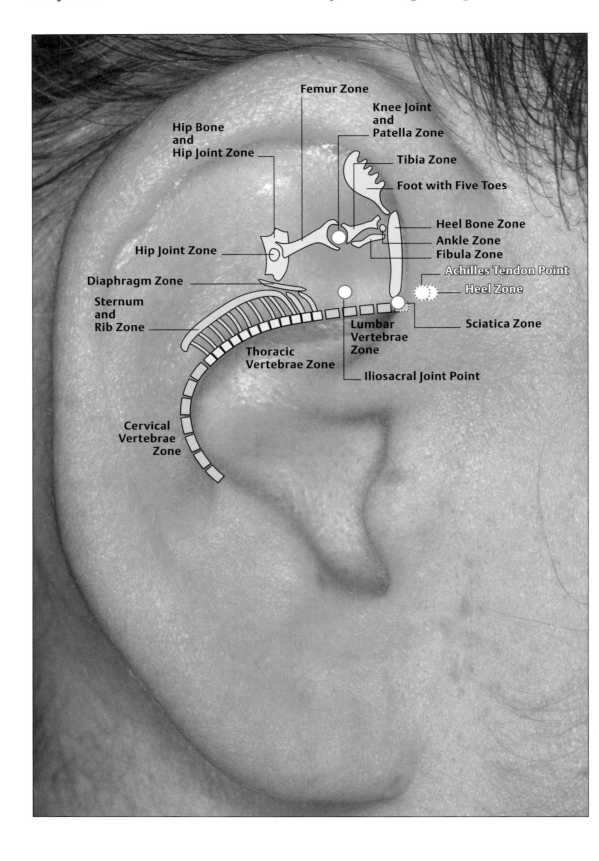

62 Finger Points

Location: In the cranial scapha, cranial to the superior anthelical crus.

Indication: Pain in the region of the fingers.

63 Clavicular Point

Location: In the scapha, roughly at the level of the supratragic notch.

Indication: Local conditions of pain (e.g. sternoclavicular obstructions).

64 Shoulder Joint Point ⊙

Location: In the scapha, roughly at the level of the lower edge of the root of helix.

Indication: Pain and afflictions in the shoulder region.

65 Shoulder Point ⊙

Location: In the scapha at the level of the elongation of the upper edge of the ascending helix branch to the helix.

Indication: Pain and afflictions in the shoulder region.

66 Elbow Point ⊙

Location: In the scapha, at the level of the inferior anthelical crus.

Indication: Pain in the elbow region.

67 Wrist Point ⊙

Location: In the scapha, at the level of the darwinian tubercle.

Indication: Pain in the wrist region.

68 Appendix Zone 1

Location: In the cranial posterior transition of the superior anthelical crus to the scapha.

Indication: No clear indications.

69 Appendix Zone 2

Location: In the scapha, at the level of an imaginary line through the inferior anthelical crus.

Indication: No clear indications.

70 Appendix Zone 3

Location: In the scapha, at the end of the helical groove.

Indication: No clear indications.

71 Urticaria Zone

Location: In the scapha, at the level of the darwinian tubercle.

Indication: Urticaria, pruritus.

For comparison:
Points on the scapha
according to Nogier *and* Bahr

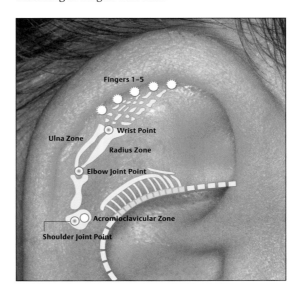

Points on the Scapha According to *Nogier*, Projection of the Upper Extremities

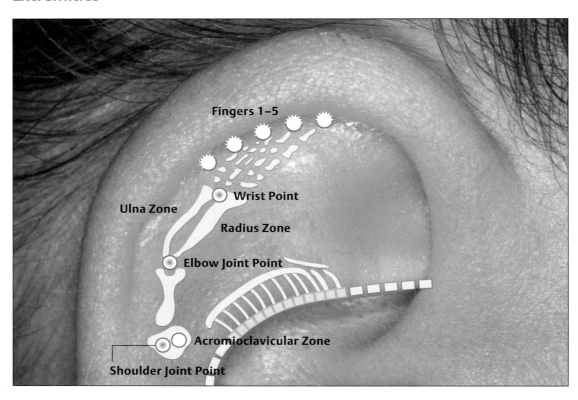

Finger Points 1–5

Location: Cranial to the wrist, partially covered by the helical rim.

Indication: Arthropathies of the finger joints.

Wrist Point ⊙

Location: In the scapha, in the area in front of the darwinian tubercle. Auxiliary line: Horizontally through the projection zone of the knee joint.

Indication: Pain in the wrist region.

Forearm Point

Location: Between the wrist and elbow joint; the radius is medial, the ulna lateral (edge of the ear).

Indication: Pain and complaints in the region of the forearm.

Elbow Joint Point ⊙

Location: In the elongation of the inferior antihelical crus to the helix in the scapha.

Indication: Pain and complaints in the elbow joint.

Upper Arm Point

Location: Between shoulder and elbow joint.

Indication: Pain and complaints in the upper arm area.

Shoulder Joint Point ⊙

Location: At the level of C7 in the scapha. C7 is located on the anthelix where the sharp fold of the cervical vertebrae changes into the soft curve of the thoracic vertebrae. Easy to detect with the stirrup sensor. C7 is located roughly in the elongation of the curve of the upper edge of the ascending helix to the cavity of concha.

Indication: Shoulder complaints, cervical vertebrae syndrome.

Acromioclavicular Joint Point

Location: At the level of C7 near the Shoulder Joint Point.

Indication: Obstructions of the acromioclavicular joint, shoulder pain.

Refresher: The most important projection zones of the upper extremity

67 (⊙) Wrist Point

66 (⊙) Elbow Point

64 (⊙) Shoulder Point

Chinese	Nogier
⊙ **67 Wrist Point** (Wrist Point)	⊙ **Wrist Point** (67 Wrist Point)
⊙ **66 Elbow Point** (Elbow Point)	⊙ **Elbow Point** (66 Elbow Point)
⊙ **64 Shoulder Point** (Shoulder Joint Point)	⊙ **Shoulder Joint Point** (64 Shoulder Point)

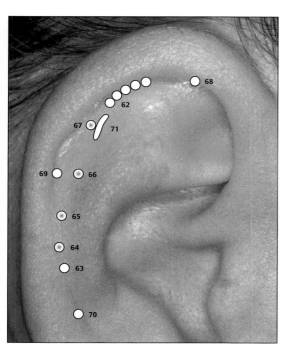

For comparison:
The projection zones of the upper extremity according to Chinese nomenclature

Topography and Indications

Points on the Scapha According to *Nogier*

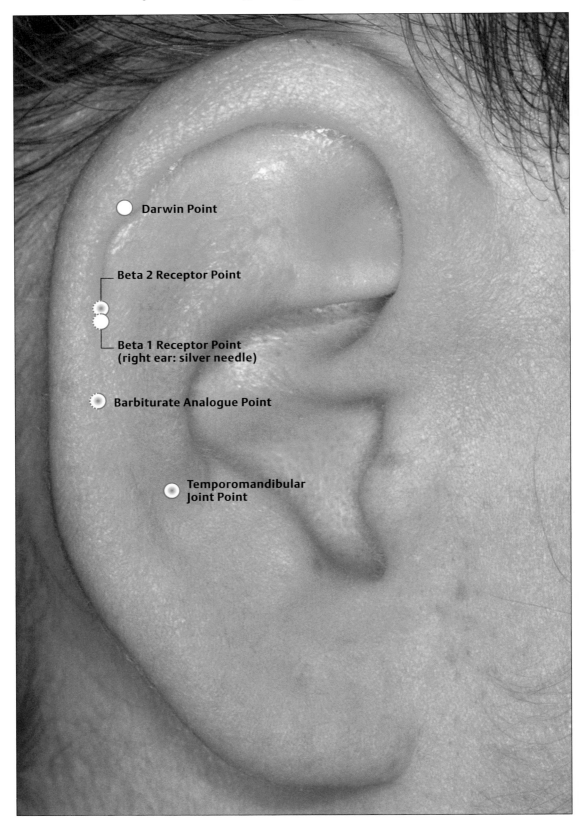

Darwin Point

Beta 2 Receptor Point

Beta 1 Receptor Point
(right ear: silver needle)

Barbiturate Analogue Point

Temporomandibular
Joint Point

Barbiturate Analogue Point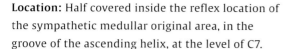

Location: Half covered inside the reflex location of the sympathetic medullar original area, in the groove of the ascending helix, at the level of C7.

Indication: Effects similar to barbiturates.

Beta 1 Receptor Point

Location: Line connecting Point Zero with T1/T2, in the helical groove.

Indication: Hypertension, beta-blocker effect.

▶ In case of right-handedness: Silver on the right, gold on the left.

Beta 2 Receptor Point

Location: Just above the Beta 1 Receptor Point.

Indication: Broncholytic effect, bronchial asthma.

▶ In case of right-handedness: Gold on the right, silver on the left.

Temporomandibular Joint Point

Location: The point is at the end of the scapha, on the postantitragal fossa.

Indication: Gnathological problems, chronic conditions of pain.

Darwin Point

Location: Darwinian tubercle.

▶ According to *Nogier*, the dividing point of innervation from the superficial cervical plexus to the trigeminal nerve.

Indication: Arthropathies of the upper and lower extremity.

Refresher: The most important points on the scapha

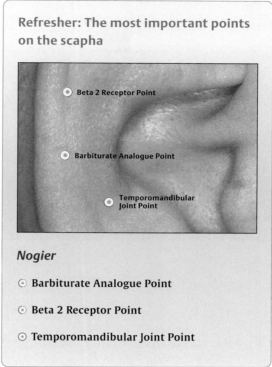

Nogier

⊙ **Barbiturate Analogue Point**

⊙ **Beta 2 Receptor Point**

⊙ **Temporomandibular Joint Point**

For comparison:
The most important points on the scapha according to Chinese nomenclature

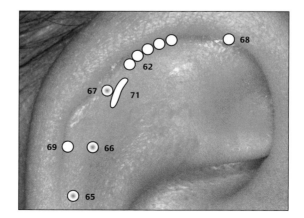

Topography and Indications

Points on the Helical Rim (Points 72–78)
According to Chinese Nomenclature and *Nogier*

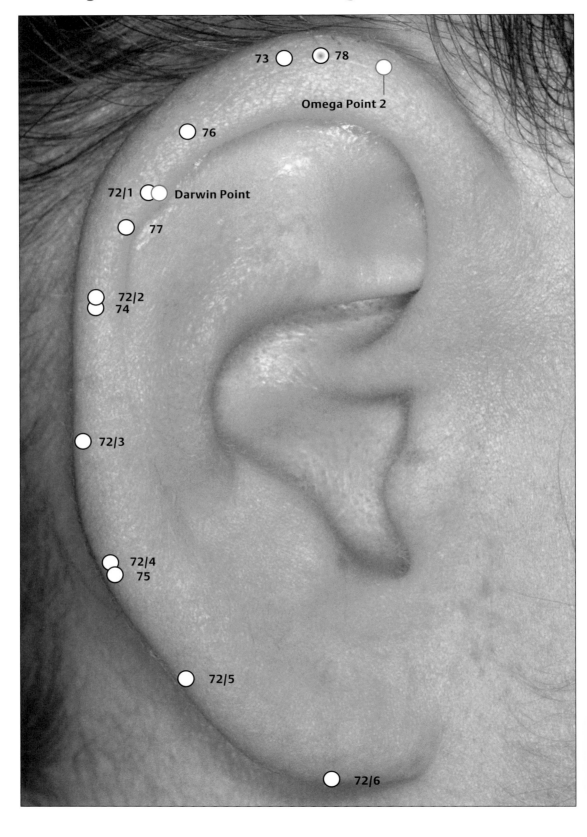

72 (1–6) Helix Point

Location: At equidistant intervals between the darwinian tubercle and the lowest point of the ear lobe.

Indication: These points provide orientation but have no therapeutic function.

73 Tonsil Point 1

Location: At the apex of the helix

Indication: As in the case of the Appendix Points, multiple projections are also involved here; general lymphatic activity (dubious).

74 Tonsil Point 2

Location: On the helix, at the level of the inferior anthelical crus.

Indication: Cf. Point 73, Tonsil Point 1.

75 Tonsil Point 3

Location: On the helix at the helix–ear lobe transition.

Indication: Cf. Point 73, Tonsil Point 1.

76 Liver Point 1

Location: Above the darwinian tubercle on the helix.

Indication: Hepatopathies.

77 Liver Point 2

Location: Below the darwinian tubercle on the helix.

Indication: Hepatopathies.

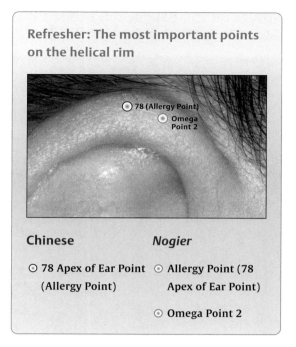

Refresher: The most important points on the helical rim

Chinese	Nogier
⊙ 78 Apex of Ear Point (Allergy Point)	⊙ Allergy Point (78 Apex of Ear Point)
	⊙ Omega Point 2

78 Apex of Ear Point ⊙
(Allergy Point According to *Nogier*)

Location: On the tip of the ear that is formed when the ear is folded over (helical rim in the direction of the crus of helix).

Indication: General modulating effect on the immune system, for example, allergies, bronchial asthma.

▶ In case of right-handedness: silver on the left.

Darwin Point

Location: Darwinian tubercle.

Indication: Arthropathies of the upper and lower extremity.

▶ According to *Nogier*, the dividing point of innervation from the superficial cervical plexus to the trigeminal nerve.

Omega Point 2

Location: On the upper edge of the helix, nasal to the Allergy Point 78.

Indication: A point of overriding importance for the motor system.

Topography and Indications

Points on the Ascending Helix Branch (Points 79–83)
According to Chinese Nomenclature

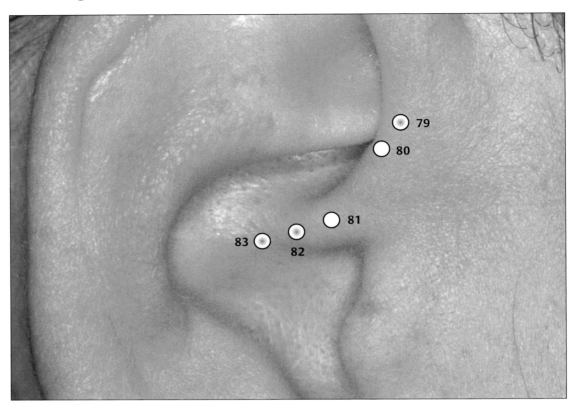

79 External Genitals Point ◉

Location: On the ascending helix branch, at the level of the inferior anthelical crus.

Indication: All forms of impotence, migraine, dysuria.

80 Urethra Point

Location: Just below the intersection of the inferior anthelical crus and the ascending helix.

Indication: Urinary tract infection, dysuria.

81 Rectum Point

Location: On the ascending helix branch, cranial to Point 82 (Diaphragm Point).

Indication: Anal complaints, hemorrhoids.

82 Diaphragm Point ◉
(Point Zero According to *Nogier*)

Location: At the intersection of the crus of helix with the ascending helix branch. Corresponds topographically to Point Zero according to *Nogier*.

Indication: Hematological disorders. The point has spasmolytic activity.

83 Bifurcation Point ⊙
(Oppression Point According to *Nogier*)

Location: At the origin of the crus of helix.

Indication: According to the Chinese school, the point does not play a major role. According to *Nogier*, End Point of the Solar Plexus Zone (Oppression Point).

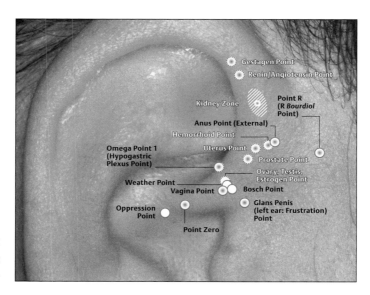

For comparison:
Points in the area of the crus of helix
according to Nogier and Bahr

Points in the Region of the Ascending Helix Branch (Crus of Helix) According to *Nogier*, External

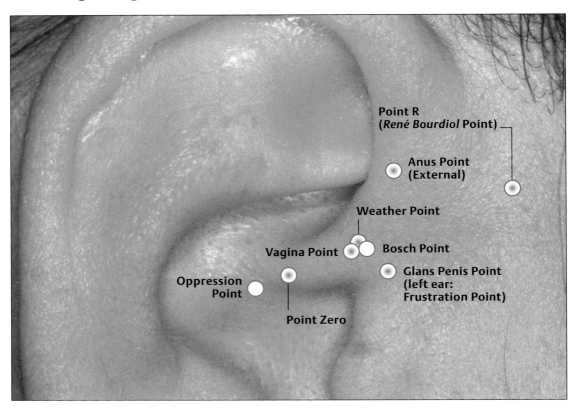

Oppression Point (Anxiety Point 2)

Location: At the origin of the crus of helix (End Point of the Solar Plexus Zone), corresponding to Point 83 (Bifurcation Point) of the Chinese school.

Indication: According to *Nogier*, End Point of the Solar Plexus. Also called "Anxiety Point." Accordingly, its indication is: Conditions of anxiety, functional gastrointestinal complaints.

Vagina Point ⊙
(According to *R. J. Bourdiol*)

Location: Cranial and lateral to the Clitoris Point.

Indication: Urogenital disorders, frigidity; pruritis vulvae.

Bosch Point (According to *Nogier*)

Location: Rim of the ascending root of helix, cranial to the supratragic notch.

Indication: An important point. Urogenital disorders, psychosomatic disorders.

Clitoris Point (According to *R. J. Bourdiol*)

Location: Corresponds to Bosch Point. *Nogier* located his Bosch Point on the lower edge of the rim.

Indication: Urogenital disorders, frigidity (cf. Bosch Point).

(External) Anus Point ⊚

Location: On the helix at the intersection with the inferior anthelical crus.

Indication: Anal complaints, anal pruritus.

Point Zero ⊚

Location: At the intersection between the crus of helix and the ascending helix branch, corresponds topographically to the location of Point 82 (Diaphragm Point) according to Chinese localization.

Indication: According to *Nogier*, this is the classic point of energy control.

- ► Treatment with gold needles in case of psychovegetative exhaustion.
  Treatment with silver needles in case of excessive needle reaction. If the ear is oversensitive, use only silver needles.

Furthermore, Point Zero has strong spasmolytic activity. In addition, hyperreflexia and hyporeflexia can be treated at this point on the auricula.

- ► Treatment with gold needles in case of hyporeflexia; with silver needles in case of hyperreflexia.

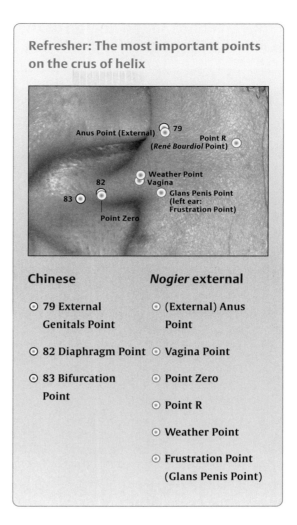

Refresher: The most important points on the crus of helix

Chinese	*Nogier* external
⊙ **79 External Genitals Point**	⊙ **(External) Anus Point**
⊙ **82 Diaphragm Point**	⊙ **Vagina Point**
⊙ **83 Bifurcation Point**	⊙ **Point Zero**
	⊙ **Point R**
	⊙ **Weather Point**
	⊙ **Frustration Point (Glans Penis Point)**

Weather Point (According to *Kropej*) ⊚

Location: In the middle of the connecting line between the supratragic notch and the intersection of the inferior anthelical crus and helix.

Indication: Sensitivity to changes in the weather. An adjuvant point for angina pectoris and migraine, often detectable on the right ear.

- ► Relative contraindication in case of pregnancy.

Point R (*René Bourdiol* Point) ⊚

Location: Elongation of the ascending helix branch, in the fossula at the transition to the face.

Indication: An adjuvant point in psychotherapy.

Frustration Point (Glans Penis Point) ⊚

Location: Toward the face on the cranial part of the supratragic notch.

- ► Right ear: Glans penis
  Left ear: Frustration

Indication: Frustration, psychosomatic disorders.

Covered Points in the Region of the Ascending Helix Branch (Crus of Helix) According to *Nogier*

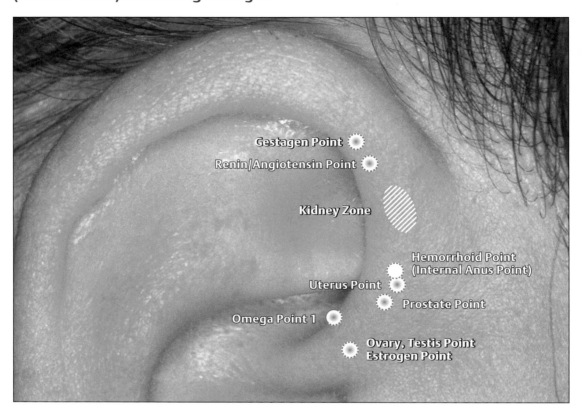

Omega Point 1
Hypogastric Plexus Point

Location: At the upper edge of the crus of helix, with the superior hemiconcha, roughly in the middle between Point Zero and the intersection between the ascending helix branch and inferior anthelical crus.

Indication: Gastrointestinal and urogenital complaints, renal colic, passing of stones (in addition, Thalamus Point and Jerome Point).
Bahr: Reference point for amalgam exposure (dominant ear in gold).

Ovary, Testis Point

Location: Slightly above the supratragic notch, on the inside (lower side) of the ascending helix, approximately 2 mm away from the reflection.

Indication: Hormonal dysfunction, hormone-related migraine.

Estrogen Point

Location: Its location corresponds to the Ovary Point.

Indication: Hormonal disorders.

Renin/Angiotensin Point

Location: Above the Renal Parenchyma Zone, on the inside, in the fold.

Indication: Arterial hypertension (treatment with silver needle on the right ear), hypotension (treatment with gold needle on the right ear).

Gestagen Point

Location: Close to the fold of the ascending helix, at the level of the superior anthelical crus.

Indication: Hormonal and menopausal complaints, hormone-related migraine.

Prostate Point

Location: Slightly above the Ovary Point, also on the inside.

Indication: Prostatis, prostate as a field of disturbance, dysuria.

Uterus Point

Location: Slightly above the Prostate Point, likewise on the inside.

Indication: Dysmenorrhea, field of disturbance after hysterectomy.

▶ Acupuncture of points influencing hormones in the area of the ascending helix is contraindicated during pregnancy.

Kidney Zone

Location: Inside the helix, roughly in the middle of the triangular fossa.

Indication: Nephropathies.

Hemorrhoid Point (Internal Anus Point)

Location: On the inside covered on the inferior anthelical crus, at the level of the intersection with the crus of helix.

Indication: Hemorrhoidal complaints, pain in the coccygeal region.

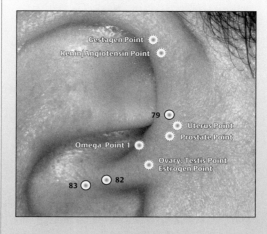

Refresher: The most important points on the crus of helix

Chinese	*Nogier* concealed
⊙ 79 External Genitals Point	⦾ Omega Point 1
⊙ 82 Diaphragm Point	⦾ Ovary, Testis Point
⊙ 83 Bifurcation Point	⦾ Estrogen Point
	⦾ Renin/Angiotensin Point
	⦾ Gestagen Point
	⦾ Prostate Point
	⦾ Uterus Point

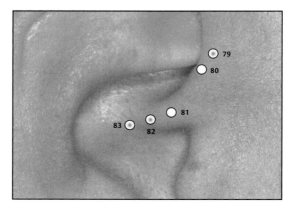

For comparison:
Points in the area of the crus of helix
according to Chinese nomenclature

Topography and Indications

Projection Zones of Internal Organs According to *R.A. Durinjan*

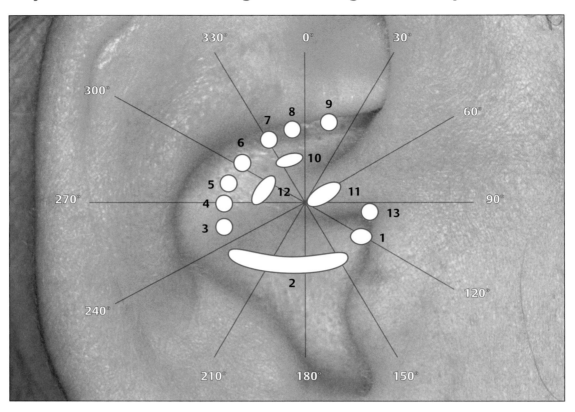

1 Tactile Taste Zone

2 Pharynx, Esophagus Zone

3 Stomach Zone

4 Duodenum Zone

5 Liver Zone

6 Gallbladder Zone

7 Pancreas Zone

8 Kidney Zone

9 Bladder Zone

10 Large Intestine Zone

11 Diaphragm Zone

12 Small Intestine Zone

13 External Genitals Zone

For comparison:
The projection zones of the internal organs
according to Nogier

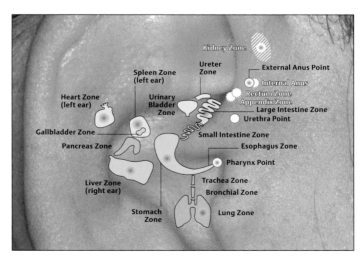

Projection Zones of Internal Organs According to Chinese Nomenclature

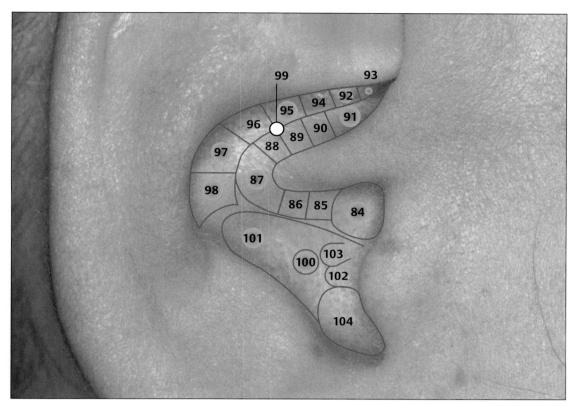

84	Mouth Zone	98	Spleen Zone
85	Esophagus Zone	99	Ascites Point
86	Cardia Zone	100	Heart Zone
87	Stomach Zone	101	Lung Zone
88	Duodenum Zone	102	Bronchial Zone
89	Small Intestine Zone	103	Trachea Zone
90	Appendix Zone 4	104	Triple Burner Zone
91	Large Intestine Zone		
92	Urinary Bladder Zone		
93	Prostate Zone		
94	Ureter Zone		
95	Kidney Zone		
96	Pancreas and Gallbladder Zone		
97	Liver Zone		

Points around the Helix Root (Points 84–91) According to Chinese Nomenclature

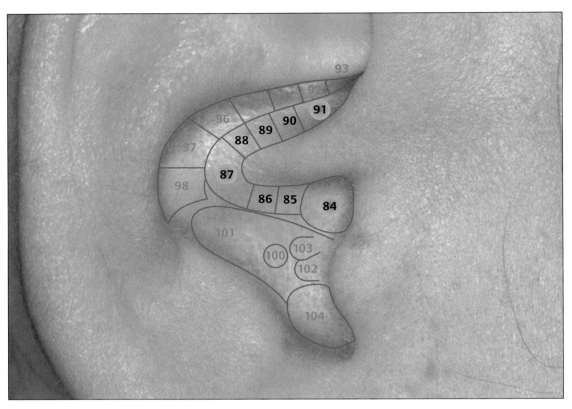

84   Mouth Zone ☉
(Thalamus Point According to *Nogier*)

Location: In the area of the supratragic notch, on the floor of the cavity of concha.

Indication: Adjuvant in addictive diseases, trigeminal neuralgia, stomatitis.

85   Esophagus Zone

Location: Caudal to the ascending root of helix on the floor of the cavity of concha, roughly in the middle.

Indication: Vomiting, difficulties swallowing, reflux.

86   Cardia Zone

Location: Lateral to Zone 85 (Esophagus Zone).

Indication: Stomach trouble, reflux.

87   Stomach Zone ☉

Location: This area surrounds the helix root and stretches into the superior cavity of concha and joins the cardia area.

Indication: Stomach disorders, nausea, vomiting, eating disturbances. Also as part of addiction treatment in weight gain or loss (e.g. during nicotine withdrawal).

88 Duodenum Zone

Location: In the superior hemiconcha next to the stomach area.

Indication: Gastrointestinal complaints.

89 Small Intestine Zone

Location: Next to Zone 88 (Duodenum Zone), cranial continuation of the digestive tract.

Indication: Gastrointestinal complaints.

90 Appendix Zone 4

Location: After the cranial continuation of Area 89 (Small Intestine Zone).

Indication: The point has lymphatic activity.

91 Large Intestine Zone ☉

Location: Cranial zone connected to Area 90 (Appendix 4), reaches to beneath the helical rim.

Indication: Gastrointestinal complaints, meteorism, constipation, diarrhea.

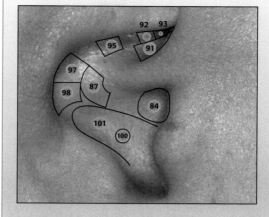

Refresher: The most important projections of the internal organs

Chinese

- ☉ **84 Mouth Zone**
- ☉ **87 Stomach Zone**
- ☉ **91 Large Intestine Zone**
- ☉ **92 Urinary Bladder Zone**
- ☉ **93 Prostate Zone**
- ☉ **95 Kidney Zone**
- ☉ **97 Liver Zone**
- ☉ **98 Spleen Zone**
- ☉ **100 Heart Zone**
- ☉ **101 Lung Zone**

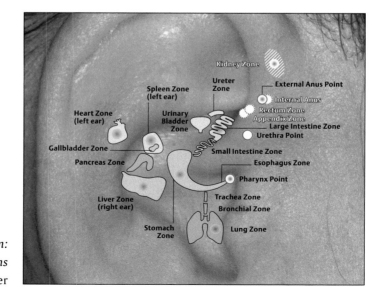

For comparison:
the projection zones of the internal organs
according to Nogier

Points in the Superior Concha (Points 92–99) According to Chinese Nomenclature

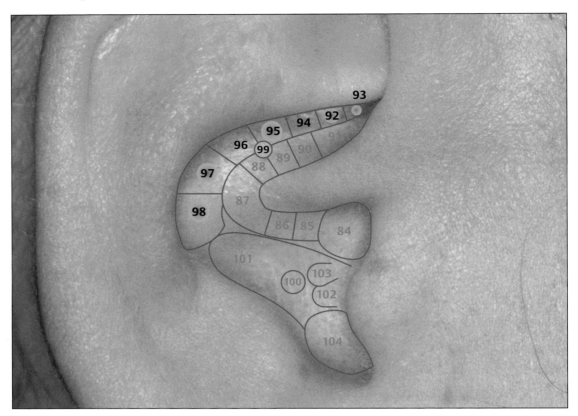

92 Urinary Bladder Zone ⊙

Location: In the part of the superior concha facing the inferior anthelical crus, above Point 91 (Large Intestine Zone).

Indication: Disorders of the urinary genital tract, dysuria, incontinence.

93 Prostate Zone ⊙

Location: In the angle formed by the crus of helix and the inferior anthelical crus, on the floor of the cavity of concha.

Indication: Disorders of the prostate, dysuria, impotence.

94 Ureter Zone

Location: Lateral to Point 92.

Indication: Dysuria.

► Often used in combination with Point 95 (Kidney Zone).

95 Kidney Zone ⊙

Location: In the middle of the superior hemiconcha.

Indication: One of the most important zones in ear acupuncture. It is used for disorders of the urogenital tract as well as joint disorders, menstrual complaints, migraine, insomnia, functional complaints, and disorders of the ear, and also for addiction treatment.

96 Pancreas and Gallbladder Zone

Location: On the edge of the ear near Area 95 (Kidney Zone) in the superior hemiconcha.

> ▶ According to Chinese localization, the gallbladder is projected on the right ear and the pancreas on the left ear. According to *Nogier*, the head of the pancreas is also projected on the right ear, while the body and tail are projected on the left ear.

Indication: Cholecystopathy, indigestion.

97 Liver Zone ⊙

Location: In the superior hemiconcha opposite the root of helix (projection zone of the stomach is projected around the root of helix).

Indication: Gastrointestinal disorders, hematological disorders, skin disorders, eye disorders. An important zone used within the scope of addiction treatment.

98 Spleen Zone ⊙

Location: Next to Area 97 (Liver Zone), reaching into the inferior hemiconcha.

> ▶ On the right ear, the liver is projected in Zones 97 and 98, while its projection on the left ear is in Zone 97.

Indication: Indigestion, hematological disorders.

99 Ascites Point

Location: Between Zones 88, 89, 95, and 96.

Indication: An adjuvant point in liver disorders.

For comparison:
The projection zones of the internal organs according to Nogier

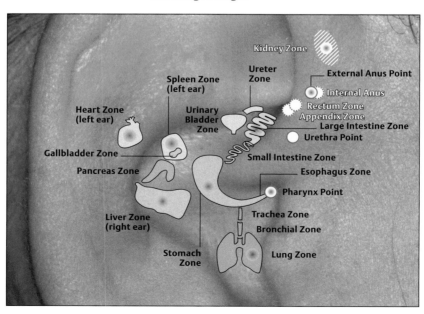

Points in the Inferior Concha (Points 100–104) According to Chinese Nomenclature

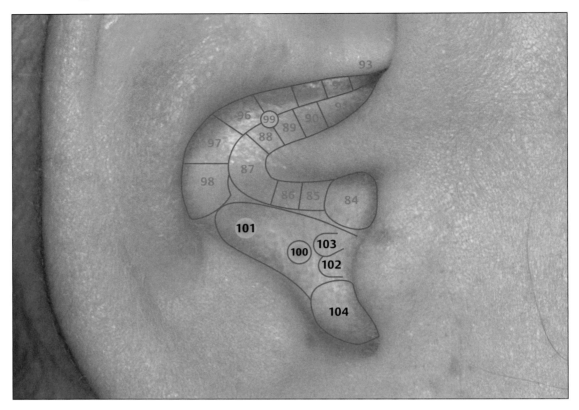

100 Heart Zone ⊙

Location: In the middle of the inferior concha.

Indication: Psychovegetative dysregulation, hypertension, hypotension, insomnia, anxiety, heart trouble, depression.

101 Lung Zone ⊙

Location: Extensive area surrounding Projection Zone 100 (Heart Zone).

Indication: Disorders of the respiratory tract, skin disorders. Used within the scope of addiction treatment, especially during nicotine withdrawal.

102 Bronchial Zone

Location: In front of the tragus in the caudal part of Zone 101 (Lung Zone).

Indication: Disorders of the respiratory tract.

103 Trachea Zone

Location: In front of the tragus in the cranial part of Zone 101 (Lung Zone).

Indication: Disorders of the respiratory tract.

104 Triple Burner Zone

Location: Caudal to Zone 101 (Lung Zone), reaching into the intertragic notch.

Indication: Gastrointestinal complaints, tendency toward edema.

Topography and Indications

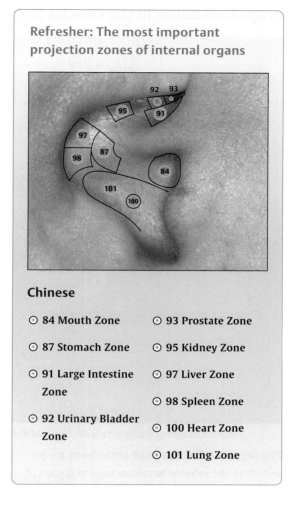

Refresher: The most important projection zones of internal organs

Chinese

- ⊙ 84 Mouth Zone
- ⊙ 87 Stomach Zone
- ⊙ 91 Large Intestine Zone
- ⊙ 92 Urinary Bladder Zone

- ⊙ 93 Prostate Zone
- ⊙ 95 Kidney Zone
- ⊙ 97 Liver Zone
- ⊙ 98 Spleen Zone
- ⊙ 100 Heart Zone
- ⊙ 101 Lung Zone

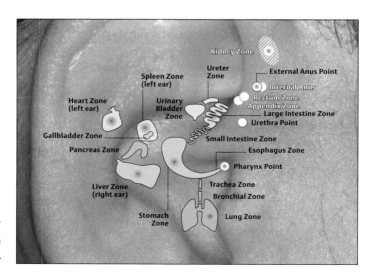

For comparison:
Points on the inferior concha
according to Nogier

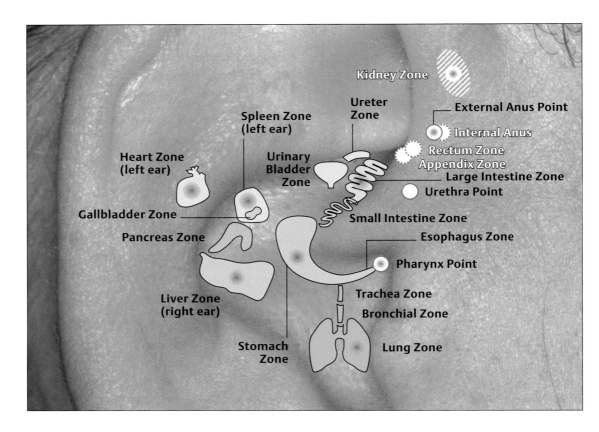

Pancreas Zone

Location: Caudal to the Gallbladder Zone in the superior hemiconcha.

The endocrine part of the pancreas is projected onto the anthelix at the level of T12 (cf. Endocrine Control Points).

Indication: Disorders of the pancreas.

Spleen Zone ⊙

Location: On the left ear, in the superior hemiconcha cranial to the Pancreas Zone.

Indication: Hematological disorders, indigestion.

Kidney Zone ⊙

Location: Covered beneath the helix, at the level of the middle of the triangular fossa.

Indication: Diseases of the kidneys.

Ureter Zone

Location: On the medial border of the Bladder Zone in the concha.

Indication: Disorders of the ureter.

Urinary Bladder Zone

Location: In the superior hemiconcha at the level of the upper lumbar vertebrae.

Indication: Diseases of the bladder.

Urethra Point

Location: On the front edge of the ascending helix where the cartilaginous border can be felt.

Indication: Disorders of the urethra.

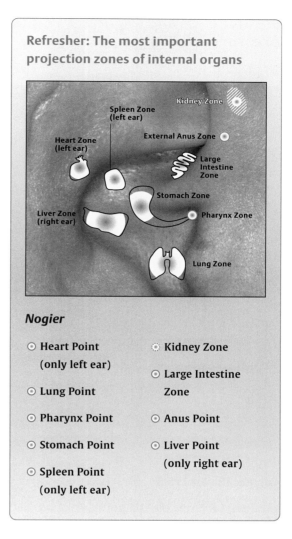

Refresher: The most important projection zones of internal organs

Nogier

- ⊙ **Heart Point** (only left ear)
- ⊙ **Lung Point**
- ⊙ **Pharynx Point**
- ⊙ **Stomach Point**
- ⊙ **Spleen Point** (only left ear)
- ☀ **Kidney Zone**
- ⊙ **Large Intestine Zone**
- ⊙ **Anus Point**
- ⊙ **Liver Point** (only right ear)

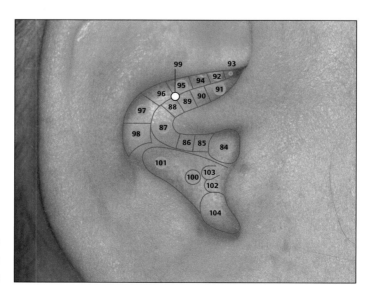

For comparison:
The projection of the internal organs
according to Chinese nomenclature

Plexus Points and Important Points in the Concha According to *Nogier*

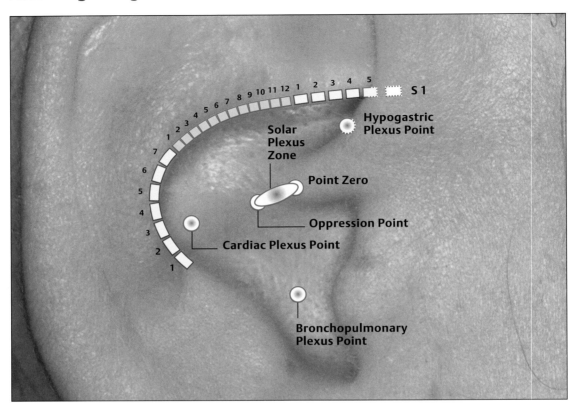

Cardiac Plexus Point ◉

Location: Ventral to the Middle Cervical Ganglion Point, at the level of C2/C3.

Indication: Hypertension, functional heart complaints, possibly in combination with Point 100 (Heart Zone).

Bronchopulmonary Plexus Point ◉

Location: In the inferior hemiconcha, roughly at the level of the peak of the tragus.

Indication: The point has broncholytic activity.

Solar Plexus Zone ◉

Location: Synonymous with Point Zero.

Indication: Gastrointestinal complaints, weakness of the so-called middle, intestinal field of disturbance, Major Energy Point (*Bahr*).

Hypogastric Plexus Point ⊙ (Omega Point 1)

Location: On the upper edge of the crus of helix, toward the superior concha, roughly in the middle between Point Zero and the intersection of the ascending helix and inferior anthelical crus.

Indication: Gastrointestinal and urogenital complaints.
Bahr: Reference point for amalgam exposure (treatment of dominant ear with gold needle).

Oppression Point (Anxiety Point 2)

Location: At the origin of the crus of helix (End Point of the Solar Plexus Zone), corresponding to Point 83 (Bifurcation Point) of the Chinese school.

Indication: According to *Nogier*, the End Point of the Solar Plexus Zone. It is also called the Anxiety Point. Accordingly, its indication is: Conditions of anxiety, functional gastrointestinal complaints.

Refresher: The most important projections on the concha

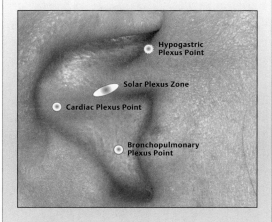

Hypogastric Plexus Point

Solar Plexus Zone

Cardiac Plexus Point

Bronchopulmonary Plexus Point

Nogier

⊙ **Bronchopulmonary Plexus Point**

⊙ **Hypogastric Plexus Point**

⊙ **Cardiac Plexus Point**

⊙ **Solar Plexus Zone**

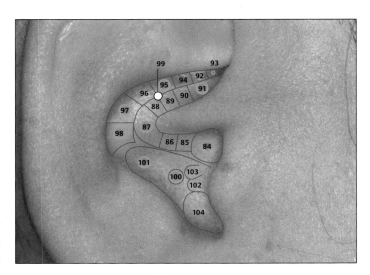

For comparison: Important points on the concha according to Chinese nomenclature

Points on the Reverse Side of the Auricula (Points 105–108) According to Chinese Nomenclature

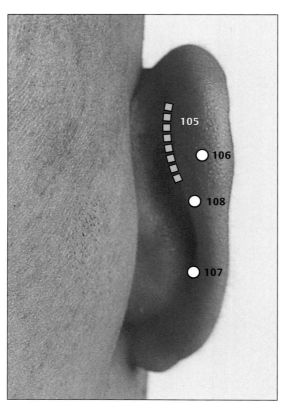

105 Blood Pressure–Reducing Furrow Zone

Location: At the beginning of the sulcus of the inferior crus.

Indication: Blood pressure reduction (bleeding).

106 Lower Back of Ear Point

Location: On the cranial edge of the superior eminence of concha, in the region of the apex of a small protuberance.

Indication: Vertebrae syndrome.

107 Upper Back of Ear Point

Location: On the upper part of the inferior eminence of concha.

Indication: Vertebrae syndrome.

108 Middle Back of Ear Point

Location: Between the projection zones of Point 106 and Point 107.

Indication: Vertebrae syndrome.

Retropoints and Projection of the Spinal Column According to *Nogier*

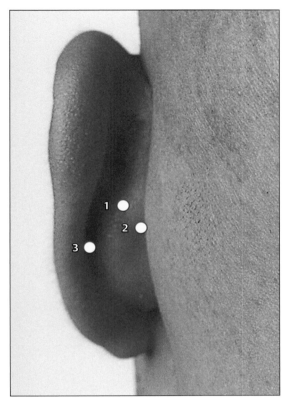
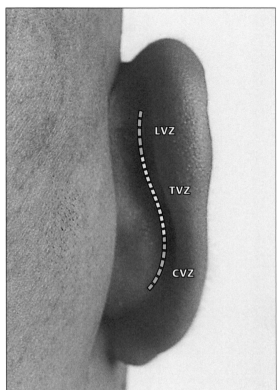

Retropoints

The significance of retropoints: The retroauricular points of the locomotor system and organs are usually projected exactly on the reverse side of the ear; the sensitive portion of the body part is mapped on the front side. The points on the diagrams should be looked at in close detail for, surprisingly, there is a slight distortion of the organ pattern so logically laid out on the front of the ear as a result of the convex form of the reverse side of the ear. While it is easy to recognize a point on the reverse side of a rubber ear by piercing it with a needle on a trial basis, this quickly becomes difficult with only a reverse representation of the ear in front of one. As on the front of the ear, the lower extremity is arranged medially to the upper extremity. But it should be noted that the Hand Point is very close to the Hip Point; the Elbow Point very close to the area of the lumbar vertebrae.

1 Retro-Point Zero

Location: In the middle of the auricula (equidistant from the upper and lower edge), approximately 0.5 cm from the point where it emerges (*Bahr*: SI-3), gold on the right side.

2 DNA Point (*Bahr*: LU-4)

3 Retro-Jerome Point

Projection Zones of the Spinal Column

LVZ Lumbar Vertebrae Zone

TVZ Thoracic Vertebrae Zone

CVZ Cervical Vertebrae Zone

Motor Points for Musculature and Joints on the Reverse Side of the Auricula According to *Nogier*

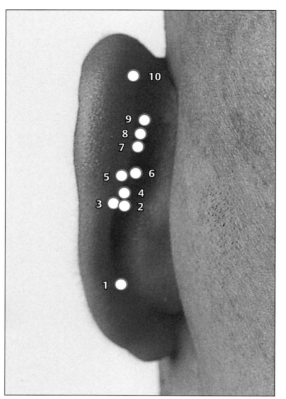 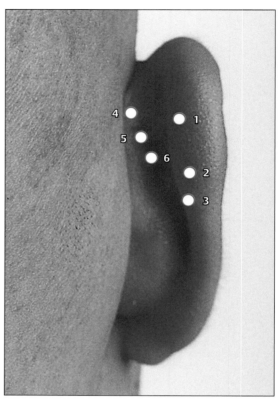

Motor Points for Musculature

1 Masseter muscle

2 Deltoideus muscle

3 Greater pectoral muscle

4 Biceps brachii muscle

5 Rectus abdominis muscle

6 Latissimus dorsi muscle

7 Greater psoas muscle

8 Gluteus maximus muscle

9 Quadriceps femoris muscle

10 Adductor pollicis muscle

Motor Points for Joints

1 Hand Point

2 Elbow Point

3 Shoulder Joint Point

4 Ankle Point

5 Knee Joint Point

6 Hip Point

Motor Points for Thorax and Abdomen on the Left and Right Ear on the Reverse Side of the Auricula According to *Nogier*

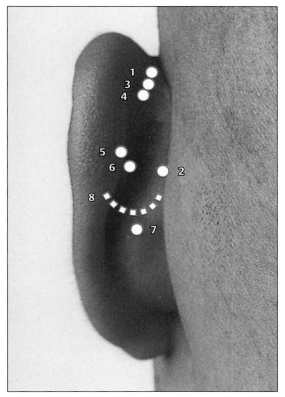

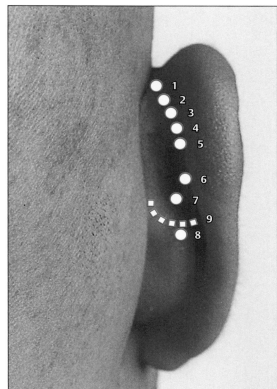

Motor Points on the Left Ear

1 Rectum Point

2 Urinary Bladder Point

3 Large Intestine Point

4 Jejunum Point

5 Heart Point

6 Stomach Point

7 Lung Point

8 Diaphragm Point (Line)

Motor Points on the Right Ear

1 Rectum Point

2 Large Intestine Point

3 Ileum Point

4 Duodenum Point

5 Gallbladder Point

6 Heart Point

7 Stomach Point

8 Lung Point

9 Diaphragm Point (Line)

Superordinate Points According to Chinese Nomenclature

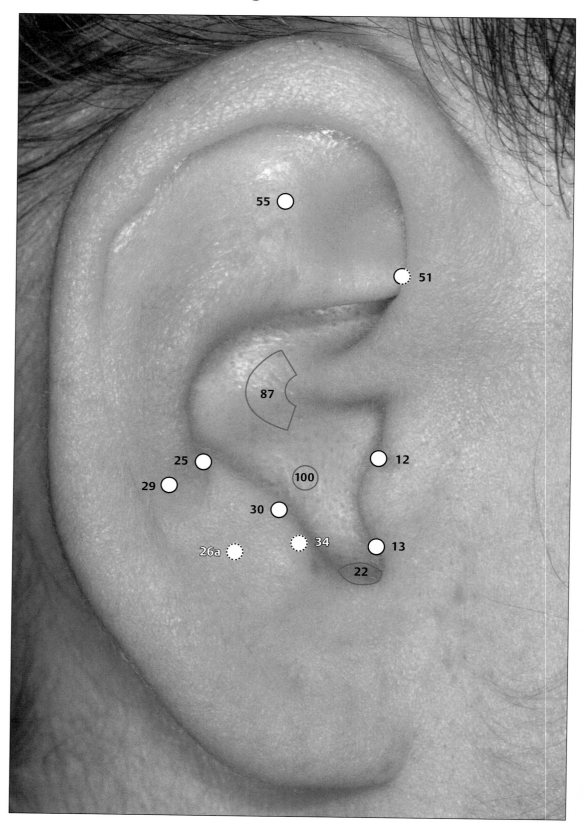

Points with Analgetic Activity

12	Apex of Tragus Point
26a	Pituitary Gland Point
29	Occiput Point
34	Gray Substance Point
55	Spirit Gate, *shen men*

Vegetative Harmonization Points

25	Brain Stem Point
29	Occiput Point
34	Gray Substance Point
51	Vegetative Point
55	Spirit Gate, *shen men*
87	Stomach Point
100	Heart Point

Points with General Antiphlogistic Activity

12	Apex of Tragus Point
13	Adrenal Gland Point
22	Endocrine Point
29	Occiput Point
34	Gray Substance Point
55	Spirit Gate, *shen men*

Antipruritic Effect

12	Apex of Tragus Point
13	Adrenal Gland Point
22	Endocrine Point
30	Parotid Gland Point

Topography and Indications

Energy and Treatment Lines on the Auricula According to *Nogier*

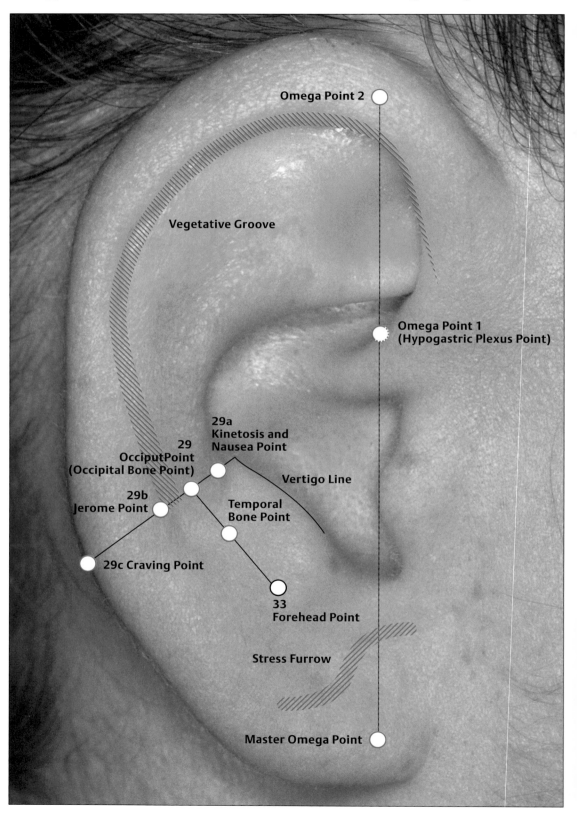

Various energy lines and treatment lines have been described on the auricula. Active acupuncture points are often found along the treatment lines. They usually form a basic framework when designing the individual treatment scheme.

Postantitragal Fossa

A straight line is drawn from Point Zero through the notch between the antitragus and anthelix and continued to the edge of the ear. Important acupuncture points are located on this line, indicated by the numbers 29a, 29, 29b, and 29c. This line is called the postantitragal fossa.

29a Kinetosis, or Nausea Point

Location: At the transition of the antitragus to the anthelix between Point 25 (Brain Stem Point, cf. p. 50) and Point 29 (Occiput Point).

Indication: Nausea, vomiting, motion sickness.

29 Occiput Point

Location: Intersection of the line connecting Point 33 (Forehead Point) and Point 35 (Sun Point) with the postantitragal fossa.

Indication: An important analgesic point, especially for cephalalgia.

29b Jerome Point (Relaxation Point)

Location: In the postantitragal fossa, at the intersection with the Vegetative Groove.

Indication: An important point with a harmonizing effect on the vegetative system in both psychosomatic disorders and sexual dysfunction.

> ► According to *Nogier*, needling of Point 29b is performed with gold needles in case of difficulty falling asleep, and with silver needles in case of difficulty staying asleep.

29c Craving Point

Location: At the end of the postantitragal fossa on the helical rim.

Indication: Psychomatic disorders and addiction treatment.

Sensory Line

Nogier calls the line between Point 33 (Forehead Point), Point 35 (Sun Point), and Point 29 (Occiput Point) the Sensory Line (p. 52). Energetic blood flow to the head is assigned to this line, as is the case with the body acupuncture points Ex-HN-3 and GV-16.

The Sensory Point described by *Nogier* lies below Point 35. As is the case with Point 35, this is used for conditions of pain as analgesic activity is also attributed to it.

The postantitragal fossa and the Sensory Line represent two basic pillars of ear acupuncture treatment. The corresponding points can be used with the associated vertebral segment for basic therapy in the treatment of conditions of pain.

Stress Furrow

This is a furrow running diagonally across the lobule. We often find it in patients who are under stress or cannot cope with stress in an appropriate manner. This furrow is of purely diagnostic importance. It has no therapeutic use.

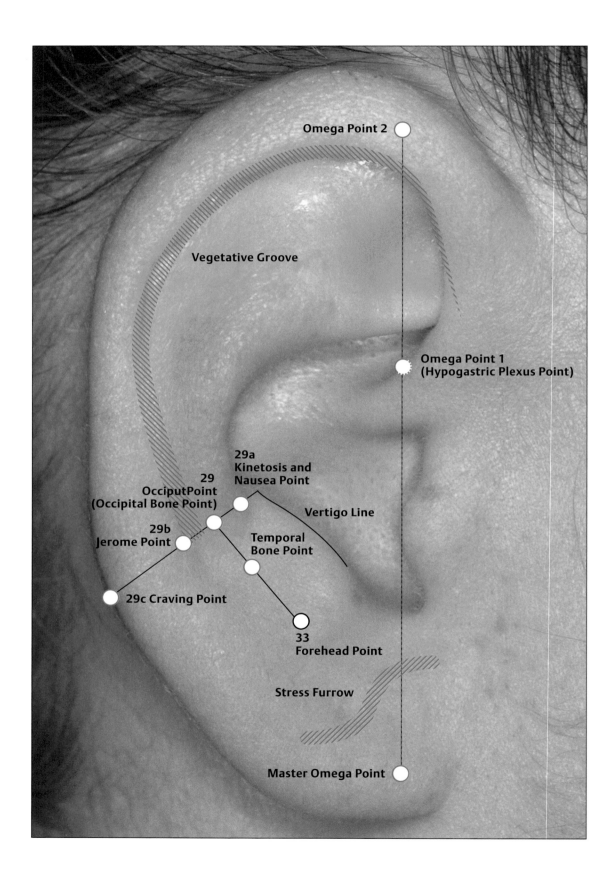

Omega Point 2

Vegetative Groove

Omega Point 1
(Hypogastric Plexus Point)

29a
Kinetosis and
Nausea Point

29
OcciputPoint
(Occipital Bone Point)

Vertigo Line

29b
Jerome Point

Temporal
Bone Point

29c Craving Point

33
Forehead Point

Stress Furrow

Master Omega Point

Line of Omega Points

This is the line connecting the three Omega Points according to *Nogier*.

Nogier divides the ear into three zones (cf. p. 6). The Entodermal Zone is assigned to metabolism, the Mesodermal Zone to the motor system, and the Ectodermal Zone to the head and central nervous system and, therefore, to a higher level of regulation.

Corresponding to this tripartition, *Nogier* found a control point for each zone.

Master Omega Point

Location: On the lower part of the lobule toward the face.

Sphere of action: Ectodermal Zone; area innervated by the cervical plexus.

Assignment: Head and central nervous system.

Omega Point 1

Location: On the upper edge of the crus of helix, in the superior hemiconcha, roughly in the middle between Point Zero and the intersection of the ascending helix and inferior anthelical crus.

Sphere of action: Entodermal Zone; area innervated by the vagus nerve.

Assignment: Metabolism.

Omega Point 2

Location: On the upper edge of the helix, nasal to the Allergy Point 78.

Sphere of action: Mesodermal Zone; area innervated by the auriculotemporal nerve of the trigeminal nerve.

Assignment: Motor system.

Vegetative Groove

The Vegetative Groove represents an important treatment tool in ear acupuncture. It should be searched for active points prior to each treatment (cf. p. 30).

Vertigo Line According to *von Steinburg*

The line runs along the postantitragal fossa and on the inside of the antitragus; it is used in case of vertigo.

Indication: Vertigo.

Needle method: One should search for the most sensitive point or points on the line.

Auxiliary Lines in Auricular Acupuncture
(B. Strittmatter)

Every ear is slightly different so that searching for points often seems difficult to the beginner. Regardless of the overall appearance of the ear relief, however, there are certain correspondences in proportion which appear to be the same for every ear. In accordance with this law, it is possible to indicate commonly applicable auxiliary lines for all shapes of ear and these make the reliable detection of several important points much easier.

This is particularly striking at the so-called axes (*Nogier/Bahr*) which pass through Point Zero: It is a never-ending source of amazement that these points actually lie on an exact line. Therefore, if two of the points are known, it is easy to infer the others (draw a line). The axis as an exceptional geometric feature has an intensifying effect on the points which are linked by it.

All metal information for needles relates to right-handed people. If a point is indicated in gold on the right, it is automatically found in silver on the left and vice versa.

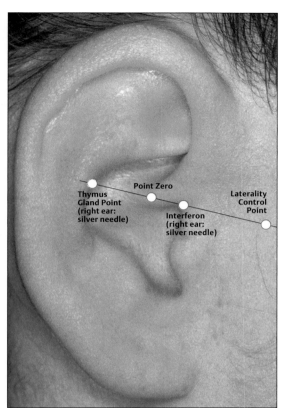

Allergy Axis 1:
Thymus Gland Point, Interferon Point, Laterality Point

The Thymus Gland Point and the Interferon Point are on a straight line through Point Zero and the Laterality Point (Thymus Gland Point in the wall at the transition of the upper third to the lower two thirds). If the axis on the left ear is needled, which is recommended, the Thymus Gland Point and the Interferon Point are gold points and the Laterality Point is a silver point.

In combination with the anti-inflammatory activity of the Interferon Point, the significance of the Thymus Gland Point, which counteracts fields of disturbance, gives this axis highly anti-allergic activity.

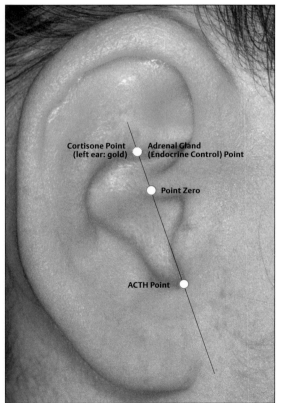

Allergy Axis 2:
Cortisone Point, ACTH Point

The Cortisone Point and ACTH Point are located on a straight line through Point Zero (Cortisone Point in the wall at the transition of the upper third to the lower two thirds, on the left in gold and on the right in silver). Therefore, if one of the two points is known, it is very easy to establish the other via the straight line through Point Zero. This axis is exceptionally effective in hay fever and allergies. Possibly in combination with Allergy Axis 1.

Antidepression Point, Tonsil Point, Temporomandibular Joint Point, Trigeminus Nerve Zone

The definition of the localization of the Antidepression Point (= Depression Point, Joy Point) is "at the end of the helical groove." The end of the helical groove may be localized very individually, however, and is often more to the cranial side. For this reason, the auxiliary line is of particular importance for the beginner so that this important symptom area or focus of irritation is not overlooked.

The straight line runs through Point Zero and the postantitragal fossa, as well as C0/C1. At the end of the scapha groove it meets the reflex localization of the Antidepression Point, Tonsil Point, retromolar area, and Temporomandibular Joint Point, which are very close to each other.

The elongation of the auxiliary line in the direction of the edge of the ear meets the Trigeminal Nerve Zone there (sensory elements on the front of the ear; motor zone on the back of the ear).

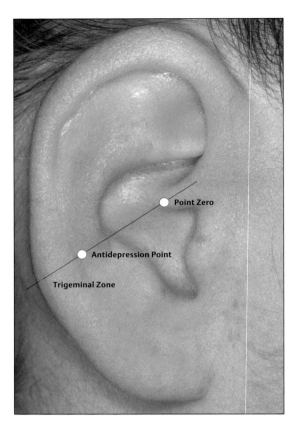

First Rib Point–Stellate Ganglion Point

The straight line between Point Zero and the point C7/T1 intersects the Stellate Ganglion Point (part of the chain of sympathetic ganglia) in the angle between the cavity of concha and the wall. The elongation via C7/T1 to the scapha touches the First Rib Point. Both points are important in inversion or in the case of a simple obstruction of the first rib.

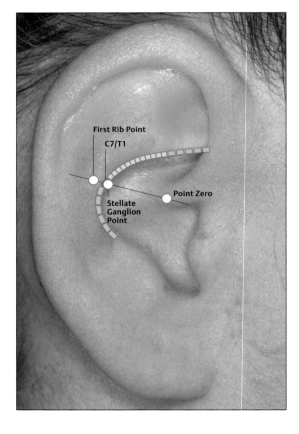

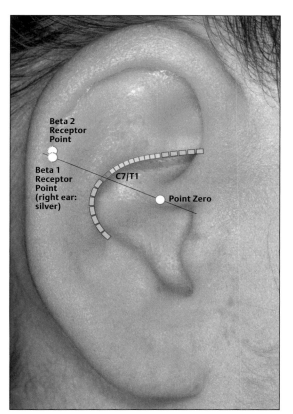

Beta 1 Receptor Point

The straight line through Point Zero and T1/T2 intersects the Beta 1 Receptor Point half-covered in the groove of the ascending helix (moderates Beta 1 receptors, reduces blood pressure; treatment on the right using silver needles). Immediately cranial to this is the Beta 2 Receptor Point (in the case of bronchospastic conditions and bronchial asthma: treatment on the right using gold needles).

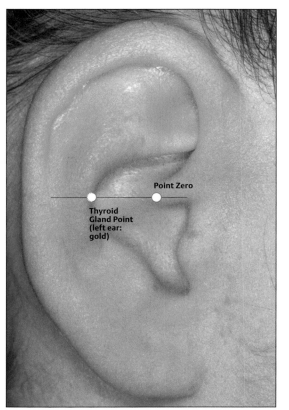

Pineal Gland Point

Horizontal line through Point Zero. If it is extended laterally, in the wall (at the transition of the upper third to the lower two thirds) it meets the reflex zone of the pineal gland in the series of endocrine organs (as a rule, treatment on the left using gold needles).

Spleen Point—Valium Point

The Spleen Point is on a straight line through Point Zero and the Valium Analogue Point on the left ear.

According to Traditional Chinese Medicine (TCM), the spleen is associated with brooding, so that combination with the Valium Point can provide very good support for vegetative harmonization.

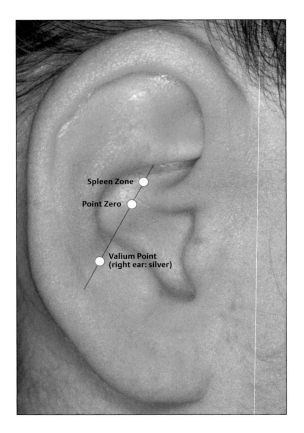

Spleen Zone

Point Zero

Valium Point
(right ear: silver)

Refresher: Comparison of the Most Important Auricular Acupuncture Points on the Left and Right Ear

As there are often difficulties with predefined localization on the right ear in finding the same point on the left ear or vice versa, the most important auricular points are once again shown in the refresher on the following pages. The corresponding points on the right and left ear are compared; in this way, localization on both ears can be achieved quickly and reliably.

Refresher: The most important points on the lobule, left ear

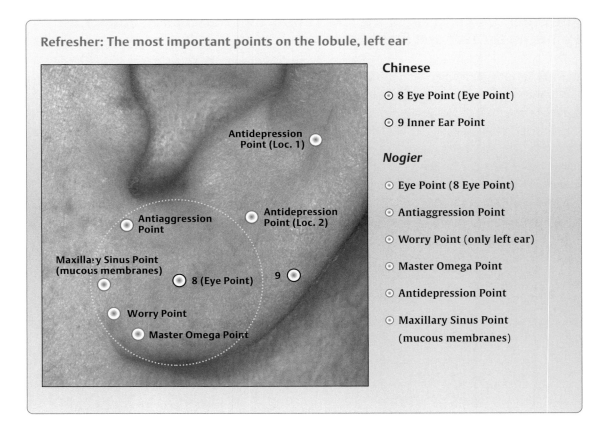

Chinese

- ◉ 8 Eye Point (Eye Point)
- ◉ 9 Inner Ear Point

Nogier

- ◉ Eye Point (8 Eye Point)
- ◉ Antiaggression Point
- ◉ Worry Point (only left ear)
- ◉ Master Omega Point
- ◉ Antidepression Point
- ◉ Maxillary Sinus Point
  (mucous membranes)

Refresher: The most important points on the tragus and supratragic notch, left ear

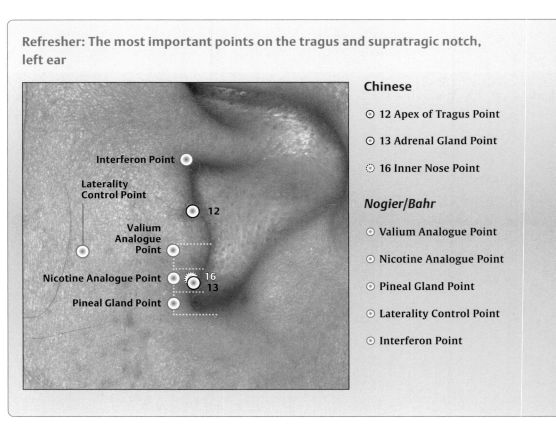

Chinese

- ◉ 12 Apex of Tragus Point
- ◉ 13 Adrenal Gland Point
- ◌ 16 Inner Nose Point

Nogier/Bahr

- ◉ Valium Analogue Point
- ◉ Nicotine Analogue Point
- ◉ Pineal Gland Point
- ◉ Laterality Control Point
- ◉ Interferon Point

Refresher: The most important points on the lobule, right ear

Chinese

⊙ 8 Eye Point (Eye Point)

⊙ 9 Inner Ear Point

Nogier

⊙ Eye Point (8 Eye Point)

⊙ Antiaggression Point

⊙ Anxiety Point (only right ear)

⊙ Master Omega Point

⊙ Antidepression Point

⊙ Maxillary Sinus Point
   (mucous membranes)

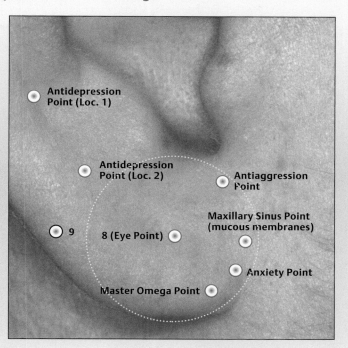

Refresher: The most important points on the tragus and supratragic notch, right ear

Chinese

⊙ 12 Apex of Tragus Point

⊙ 13 Adrenal Gland Point

⊙ 16 Inner Nose Point

Nogier

⊙ Valium Analogue Point

⊙ Nicotine Analogue Point

⊙ Pineal Gland Point

⊙ Laterality Control Point

⊙ Interferon Point

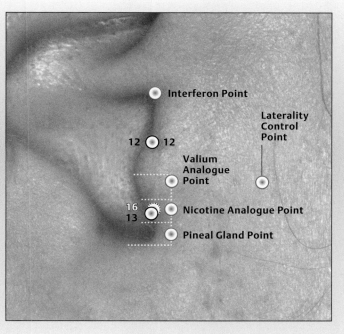

Refresher: The most important points on the intertragic notch, left ear

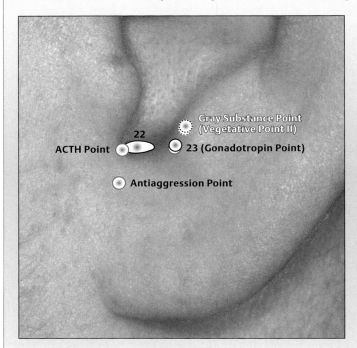

Chinese

- ⊙ 22 Endocrine Point
- ⊙ 23 Ovary Point
  (Gonadotropin Point)
- ⊙ 34 Gray Substance Point
  (Vegetative Point II)

Nogier

- ⊙ Antiaggression Point
- ⊙ Gonadotropin Point
  (23 Ovary Point)
- ⊙ ACTH Point
- ⊙ Vegetative Point II
  (34 Gray Substance Point)

Refresher: The most important points on the antitragus, left ear

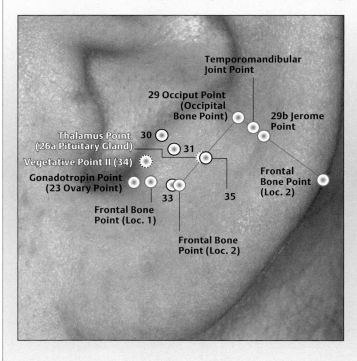

Chinese

- ⊙ 23 Ovary Point
  (Gonadotropin Point)
- ⊙ 26a Pituitary Gland Point
  (Thalamus)
- ⊙ 29 Epithelium Point
  (Occipital Bone Point)
- ⊙ 30 Parotis
- ⊙ 31 Asthma
- ⊙ 33 Forehead (Os frontale)
- ⊙ 34 Gray Substance Point
  (Vegetative Point II)
- ⊙ 35 Sun Point (Os temporale)

► Contin.

Refresher: The most important points on the intertragic notch, right ear

Chinese

⊙ 22 Endocrine Point

⊙ 23 Ovary Point
(Gonadotropin Point)

⊙ 34 Gray Substance Point
(Vegetative Point II)

Nogier

⊙ Antiaggression Point

⊙ Gonadotropin Point
(23 Ovary Point)

⊙ ACTH Point

⊙ Vegetative Point II
(34 Gray Substance Point)

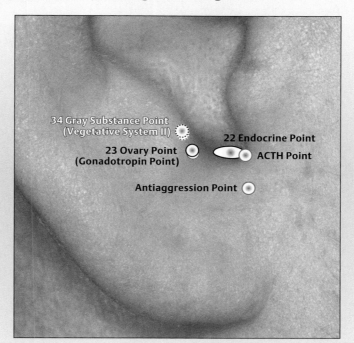

Refresher: The most important points on the antitragus, right ear

► Contin.

Nogier/Bahr

⊙ Occipital Bone Point
(29 Epithelium Point)

⊙ 29b Jerome Point

⊙ 29c Craving Point

⊙ Vegetative Point II
(34 Gray Substance Point)

⊙ Thalamus
(26a Pituitary Gland Point)

⊙ Gonadotropin Point
(23 Ovary Point)

⊙ Temporomandibular Joint Point

⊙ Frontal Bone Point
(33 Forehead Point)

⊙ Temporal Bone Point
(35 Sun Point)

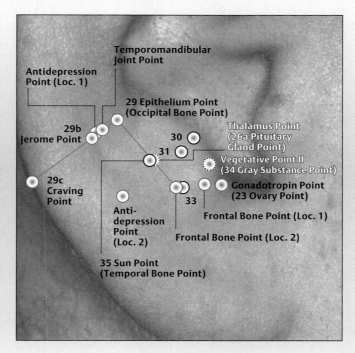

Refresher: The most important points on the superior and inferior anthelical crura, left ear

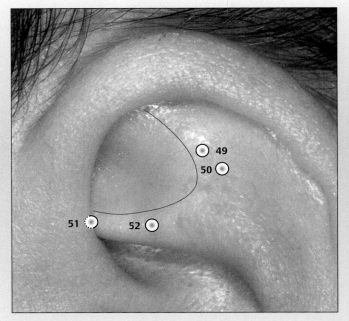

Chinese

⊙ 49 Knee Joint Point

⊙ 50 Hip Point

⊙ 51 Vegetative Point

⊙ 52 Sciatic Nerve Point

Nogier

According to *Nogier* the projection zones for the lower extremity are on the triangular fossa.

Refresher: The most important points on the triangular fossa, left ear

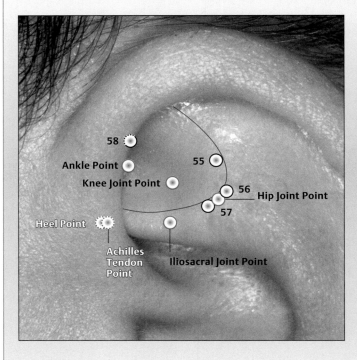

Chinese

⊙ 55 *shen men*

⊙ 56 Pelvis Point

⊙ 57 Hip Point

⊙ 58 Uterus Point

Nogier

⊙ Hip Joint Point

⊙ Ankle Point

⊙ Knee Joint Point

⊙ Achilles Tendon Point

⊙ Heel Point

⊙ Iliosacral Joint Point

Refresher: The most important points on the superior and inferior anthelical crura, right ear

Chinese

- ⊙ 49 Knee Joint Point
- ⊙ 50 Hip Point
- ⊛ 51 Vegetative Point
- ⊙ 52 Sciatic Nerve Point

Nogier

According to *Nogier* the projection zones for the lower extremity are on the triangular fossa.

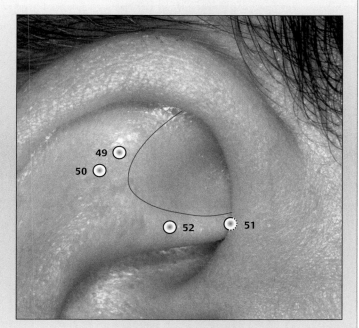

Refresher: The most important points on the triangular fossa, right ear

Chinese

- ⊛ 55 *shen men*
- ⊙ 56 Pelvis Point
- ⊙ 57 Hip Point
- ⊙ 58 Uterus Point

Nogier

- ⊙ Hip Joint Point
- ⊙ Ankle Point
- ⊙ Knee Joint Point
- ⊛ Achilles Tendon Point
- ⊛ Heel Point
- ⊙ Iliosacral Joint Point

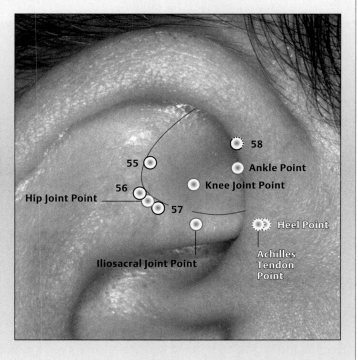

Refresher: The most important points of the upper extremity on the scapha, left ear

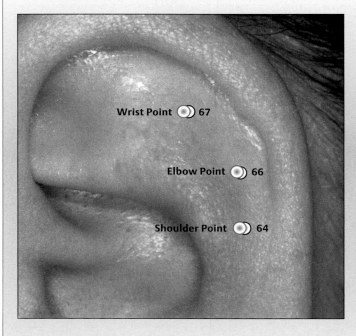

Chinese

⊙ 67 Wrist Point
(Wrist Joint Point)

⊙ 66 Elbow Point
(Elbow Joint Point)

⊙ 64 Shoulder Point
(Shoulder Joint Point)

Nogier

⊙ Wrist Joint Point (67 Wrist Point)

⊙ Elbow Joint Point
(66 Elbow Point)

⊙ Shoulder Joint Point
(64 Shoulder Point)

Refresher: The most important points on the scapha, left ear

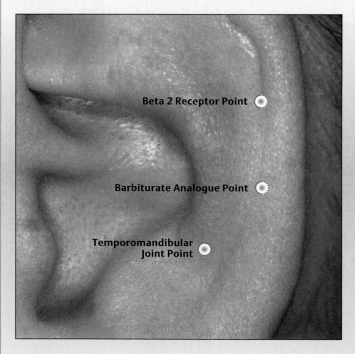

Nogier

⊙ Barbiturate Analogue Point

⊙ Beta 2 Receptor Point

⊙ Temporomandibular Joint Point

Refresher: The most important points of the upper extremity on the scapha, right ear

Chinese

⊙ 67 Wrist Point
(Wrist Joint Point)

⊙ 66 Elbow Point
(Elbow Joint Point)

⊙ 64 Shoulder Point
(Shoulder Joint Point)

Nogier

⊙ Wrist Joint Point (67 Wrist Point)

⊙ Elbow Joint Point
(66 Elbow Point)

⊙ Shoulder Joint Point
(64 Shoulder Point)

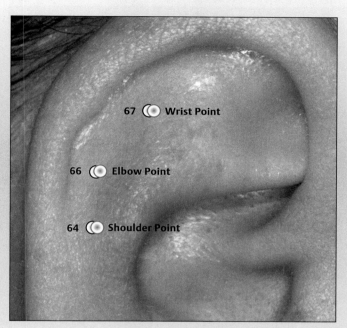

Refresher: The most important points on the scapha, right ear

Nogier

⊙ Barbiturate Analogue Point

⊙ Beta 2 Receptor Point

⊙ Temporomandibular Joint Point

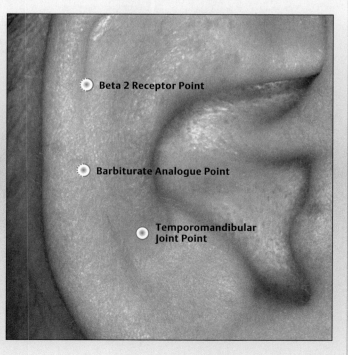

Refresher: The most important points on the helical rim, left ear

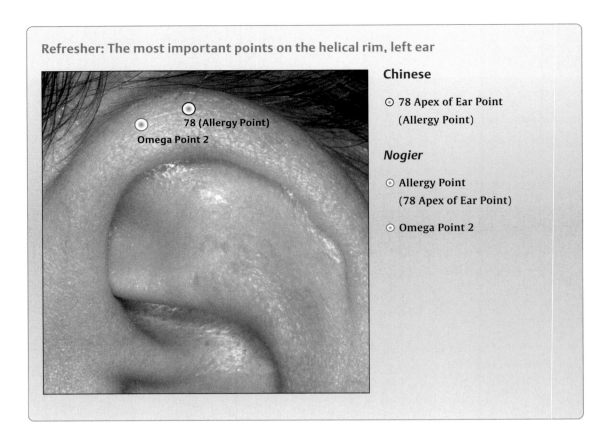

Chinese

- ☉ 78 Apex of Ear Point
  (Allergy Point)

Nogier

- ☉ Allergy Point
  (78 Apex of Ear Point)
- ☉ Omega Point 2

Refresher: The most important points on the crus of helix, left ear

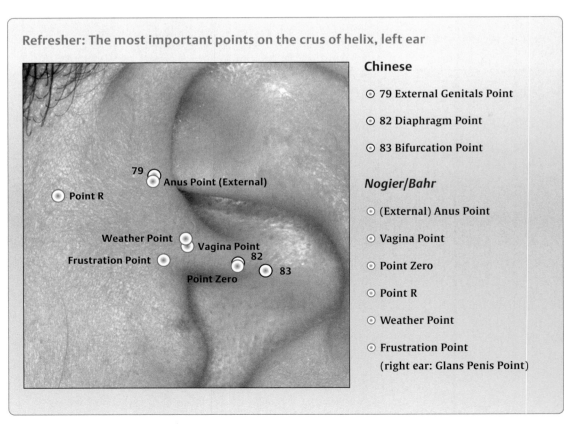

Chinese

- ☉ 79 External Genitals Point
- ☉ 82 Diaphragm Point
- ☉ 83 Bifurcation Point

Nogier/Bahr

- ☉ (External) Anus Point
- ☉ Vagina Point
- ☉ Point Zero
- ☉ Point R
- ☉ Weather Point
- ☉ Frustration Point
  (right ear: Glans Penis Point)

Refresher: The most important projection zones of internal organs according to *Nogier*, right ear

Nogier

- ⊙ Lung Zone
- ⊙ Pharynx Zone
- ⊙ Stomach Zone
- ⊙ Kidney Zone
- ⊙ Large Intestine Zone
- ⊙ Anus Zone
- ⊙ Liver Zone (only right ear)

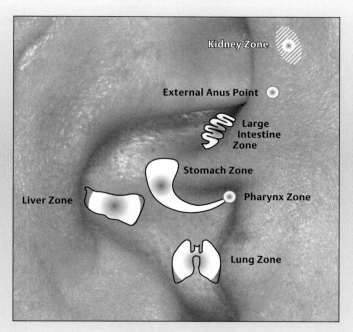

Refresher: The most important plexus points on the concha, right ear

Nogier

- ⊙ Bronchopulmonary Plexus Point
- ⊙ Cardiac Plexus Point
- ⊙ Hypogastric Plexus Point
- ⊙ Solar Plexus Point

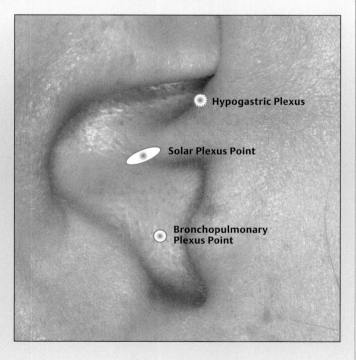

3 Treatment of Major Illnesses

*(H.-U. Hecker, D. Mühlhoff, A. Steveling,
E.T. Peuker, K.-H. Junghanns †)*

Antidepression Point (Loc. 1)

Trigeminal Zone (Loc. 1)

Antidepression Point (Loc. 2)

Antiaggression Point

Trigeminal Zone (Loc. 2)

Eye Point

Joy (left ear: Sorrow) Point

Introduction

Set out below are examples of treatments for major illnesses encountered in everyday practice and which respond to auricular acupuncture. These examples take into account points according to the Chinese school and points according to *Nogier*.

To a far greater extent than body acupuncture, auricular acupuncture is a mixture of points

1. which are taken pragmatically from the micro-somatope,

2. which comply with the theory of Traditional Chinese Medicine (TCM), and

3. which arise from pathophysiological, orthodox Western medical theories. (Point selection according to Chinese criteria has already been referred to on p. 32.)

The beginner will initially restrict himself/herself to the points of the somatope (a lung disease is treated via the Lung Point; a disease of the Lumbar Vertebrae Zone [LVZ] is treated in the LVZ section in the auricula) and to the points according to Western pathophysiological findings (an allergic illness is treated via the ACTH Point or the Adrenal Gland Point to exert an influence on glucocorticoid metabolism or to promote adrenergic hormonal influence).

From a traditional Chinese viewpoint, the advanced student will select points which relate, for example, to the Theory of Five Elements. Thus, arterial hypertension can be treated pragmatically in the blood pressure–reduction furrow but, according to the TCM perspective, regulated via the Liver Point (stores the blood, regulates excessive liver *yang*) and Heart Point (moves the blood).

The selection of *Nogier* points is always individual to the patient depending on the acute findings (active auricular acupuncture points). Experience shows that the additional auricular acupuncture points specified according to *Nogier* can frequently be found as active auricular acupuncture points in the corresponding illnesses. However, it should be pointed out once again that auricular acupuncture points should not be used rigidly according to pre-determined point combinations but according to the examination findings based on active points.

Nonetheless, it is a useful aid for the beginner to use the predetermined points as a guide.

Internal and Psychosomatic Disorders
(D. Mühlhoff, H.-U. Hecker)

Acupuncture or auricular acupuncture can be a supportive treatment option in treating psychosomatic illnesses. Fixed treatment programs cannot be specified, though. The corresponding complaints form the basis for point selection, with individual circumstances being taken into account.

Treatment of Pollinosis

Points According to Chinese Nomenclature

13   Adrenal Gland Point
14   External Nose Point
16   Inner Nose Point
22   Endocrine Point
23   Ovary Point
30   Parotid Gland Point
51   Vegetative Point
55   *Shen men*
71   Urticaria Zone
78   Apex of Ear Point
100 Heart Zone
101 Lung Zone
102 Bronchial Zone
103 Trachea Zone

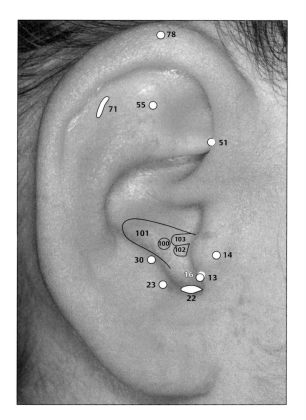

Points According to *Nogier* and *Bahr*

Allergy Point (= Chinese Point 78 [Apex of Ear Point], possibly microphlebotomy)
Nose Point
Sneezing Point
Occiput Point
Interferon Point
Thymus Gland Point
ACTH Point

► Here, combination with body acupuncture has in particular proved its worth. A basic formula in the treatment of pollinosis via body acupuncture are the points LI-4, LI-11, Ex-HN-1, BL-2, LI-20.

► Retuning of the immune system as part of the treatment of pollinosis is useful. This can be done with small amounts of the patient's own blood (up to 0.5 mL). The addition of a homeopathic retuning remedy such as Formic Acid D 6 has also proved worthwhile.

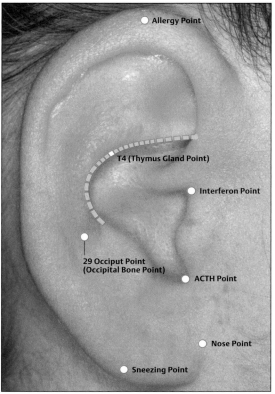

Diseases of the Respiratory Tract

Points According to Chinese Nomenclature

12   Apex of Tragus Point
13   Adrenal Gland Point
15   Larynx Point
16   Inner Nose Point
22   Endocrine Point
31   Asthma Point
42   Thorax Point
51   Vegetative Point
55   *Shen men*
60   Dyspnea Point
91   Large Intestine Point
95   Kidney, Adrenal Gland Point (functional)
101 Lung Zone
102 Bronchial Zone

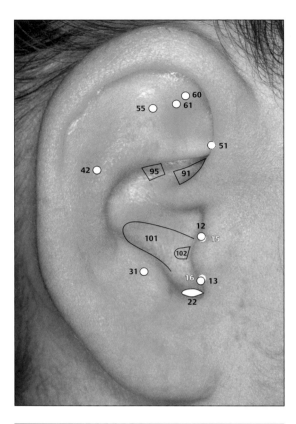

Points According to *Nogier* and *Bahr*

Bronchopulmonary Plexus Point
Point Zero
Stellate Ganglion Point
ACTH Point
Thymus Gland Point
Interferon Point
Allergy Point (= Chinese Point 78 [Apex of Ear Point])
Beta 2 Receptor Point
Occiput Point
Temporomandibular Joint Point
Omega Points
Thalamus Point

► The irritated vertebral segment located in the region of the Cervical Vertebrae Zone (CVZ), the Thoracic Vertebrae Zone (TVZ) or—seldom—the LVZ should be included in the treatment.

► We find the irritated segment with the aid of the point searching device or the anatomical condition (scaling, pressure sensitivity, etc.). Based on this, additional treatment points can be found (cf. p. 30).

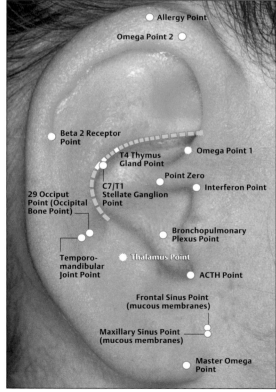

Frequently Found Point Combinations in Disorders of the Respiratory Tract

Asthma

22 Endocrine Point
31 Asthma Point
51 Vegetative Point
55 *Shen men*
60 Dyspnea Point
101 Lung Zone
....
Allergy Point
ACTH Point
Thymus Gland Point
Irritated Vertebral Segment Point
Stellate Ganglion Point
Frontal Sinus Point (mucous membranes)
Maxillary Sinus Point (mucous membranes)

Bronchitis

13 Adrenal Gland Point
29 Occiput Point
51 Vegetative Point
55 *Shen men*
101 Lung Zone
102 Bronchial Zone

Sinusitis

13 Adrenal Gland Point
16 Inner Nose Point
22 Endocrine Point
101 Lung Zone
....
Frontal Sinus Point (mucous membranes)
Maxillary Sinus Point (mucous membranes)
ACTH Point
Allergy Point
Frontal Bone Point

Allergic Rhinitis

13 Adrenal Gland Point
16 Inner Nose Point
22 Endocrine Point
23 Ovary Point
....
Allergy Point
ACTH Point

Rhinitis sicca

13 Adrenal Gland Point
16 Inner Nose Point
33 Forehead Point
98 Spleen Zone
101 Lung Zone
....
Frontal Sinus Point (mucous membranes)
Maxillary Sinus Point (mucous membranes)

Pain in the Chest

29 Occiput Point
42 Thorax Point
55 *Shen men*
101 Lung Zone
....
First Rib Point
Stellate Ganglion Point
Irritated Vertebral Segment Point
Temporomandibular Joint Point

Cardiovascular Diseases

Points According to Chinese Nomenclature

13 Adrenal Gland Point
19 Hypertonus Point
34 Gray Substance Point
51 Vegetative Point
55 *Shen men*
59 Blood Pressure–Reduction Point
95 Kidney, Adrenal Gland Point (functional)
97 Liver Zone
98 Spleen Zone
100 Heart Zone
105 Blood Pressure–Reduction Furrow (rear side of the auricula, cf. p. 135)

Points According to *Nogier* and *Bahr*

Thalamus Point

> ► According to *Nogier*, blood pressure is reduced by means of a gold needle and raised by means of a silver needle.

Master Omega Point
Antiaggression Point
29b Jerome Point
Cardiac Plexus Point
Point Zero
Beta 1 Receptor Point
Renin/Angiotensin Point
Irritated Vertebral Segment Point
First Rib Point
Stellate Ganglion Point
Heart Point

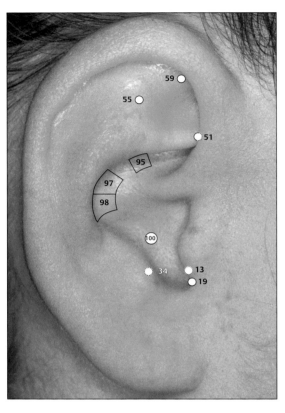

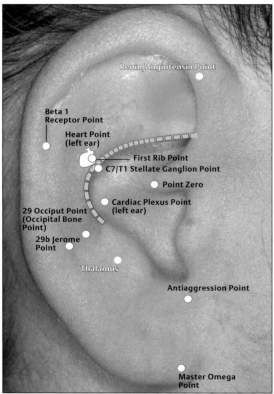

Frequently Found Point Combinations in Diseases of the Cardiovascular System

► Life-threatening diseases represent a contraindication for acupuncture. In diseases such as, for example, malignant heart rhythm disturbances or angina pectoris, acupuncture can only provide support.

Hypertension

19 Hypertension Point
51 Vegetative Point
55 *Shen men*
95 Kidney Zone
97 Liver Zone
100 Heart Point
....
Antiaggression Point
Cardiac Plexus Point
29b Jerome Point
Beta 1 Receptor Point
Thalamus Point
Renin/Angiotensin Point

Hypotension

13 Adrenal Gland Point
34 Gray Substance Point
100 Heart Point
....
Renin/Angiotensin Point
Heart Point

Heart Rhythm Disturbances

29 Occiput Point
29b Jerome Point
51 Vegetative Point
55 *Shen men*
100 Heart Point
....
Irritated Vertebral Segment Point
Stellate Ganglion Point
First Rib Point
Antiaggression Point
Cardiac Plexus Point

Angina Pectoris

42 Thorax Point
51 Vegetative Point
55 *Shen men*
100 Heart Point
....
Irritated Vertebral Segment Point
29 Occiput Point

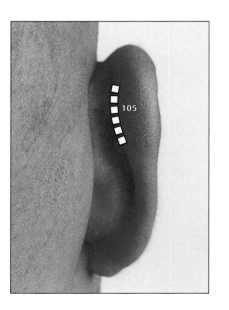

Diseases of the Digestive Organs

Points According to Chinese Nomenclature

9   Inner Ear Point
22   Endocrine Point
34   Gray Substance Point
51   Vegetative Point
55   *Shen men*
81   Rectum Point
82   Diaphragm Point
85   Esophagus Point
86   Cardia
87   Stomach Point
88   Duodenum Point
89   Small Intestine Point
91   Large Intestine Point
96   Pancreas and Gallbladder Zone
97   Liver Zone
98   Spleen Zone
100   Heart Zone

Points According to *Nogier*

Irritated Vertebral Segment Point
Antiaggression Point
29 Occiput Point
29a Kinetosis and Nausea Point
29b Jerome Point
Diaphragm Point
Solar Plexus Zone
Anxiety Point
Vegetative Point II
Hypogastric Plexus Point (= Omega 1)
Anus Point (External and Internal)
Oppression Point (= Anxiety Point 2)
Allergy Point
Zones of corresponding internal organs
ACTH Point

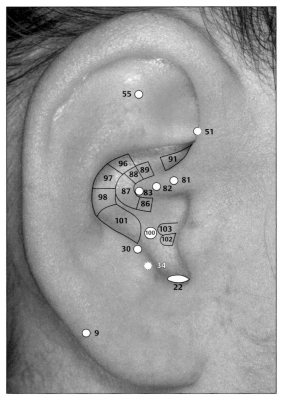

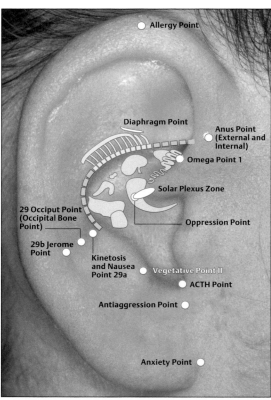

Frequently Found Point Combinations in Diseases of the Digestive Organs

Functional Gastrointestinal Complaints

51 Vegetative Point
55 *Shen men*
87 Stomach Point
89 Small Intestine Point
91 Large Intestine Point
100 Heart Zone
....
29 Occiput Point
29b Jerome Point
Antiaggression Point

Nausea, Sickness

9 Inner Ear Point
29 Occiput Point
51 Vegetative Point
55 *Shen men*
82 Diaphragm Point
87 Stomach Point
....
29a Kinetosis and Nausea Point
Diaphragm Point
Solar Plexus Zone

Colic-like Complaints

51 Vegetative Point
55 *Shen men*
82 Diaphragm Point
89 Small Intestine Point
91 Large Intestine Point
....
Hypogastric Plexus Point
Irritated Vertebral Segment Point
29b Jerome Point
Diaphragm Point

Singultus

34 Gray Substance Point
51 Vegetative Point
55 *Shen men*
82 Diaphragm Point
....
Irritated Vertebral Segment Point
Diaphragm Point

Dyspepsia

22 Endocrine Point
89 Small Intestine Point
97 Liver Zone
98 Spleen Zone

Anal Pruritus

22 Endocrine Point
30 Parotid Gland Point
34 Gray Substance Point
....
Allergy Point
Anus Point
   (External and Internal)
Rectum Point
Hemorrhoid Point
ACTH Point
Antiaggression Point

Colitis

29 Occiput Point
34 Gray Substance Point
55 *Shen men*
87 Stomach Point
89 Small Intestine Point
91 Large Intestine Point
100 Heart Zone
....
Allergy Point
ACTH Point
Antiaggression Point
Oppression Point
Vegetative Point II

Constipation

55 *Shen men*
81 Rectum Point
89 Small Intestine Point
91 Large Intestine Point

Diarrhea

55 *Shen men*
89 Small Intestine Point
91 Large Intestine Point
98 Spleen Zone

Psychosomatic Disorders

Points According to Chinese Nomenclature

25   Brain Stem Point
26a Pituitary Gland Point
34   Gray Substance Point
51   Vegetative Point
55   *Shen men*
100 Heart Point

Points According to *Nogier* and *Bahr*

Vegetative Point II
Points on the postantitragal fossa
(Line: Point 29a, Kinetosis and Nausea Point—Point
29, Occiput Point—Point 29b, Jerome Point—Point
29c, Craving Point)
Antidepression Point
Antiaggression Point
Anxiety Point
Anxiety Point 2 (Oppression Point)
Joy Point, Sorrow Point
Omega Points (1, 2, Master Point)
Point R (according to *R.J. Bourdiol*)
Thalamus Point (= Chinese 26a [Pituitary Gland
Point])
Valium Analogue Point
Barbiturate Analogue Point
Frustration Point

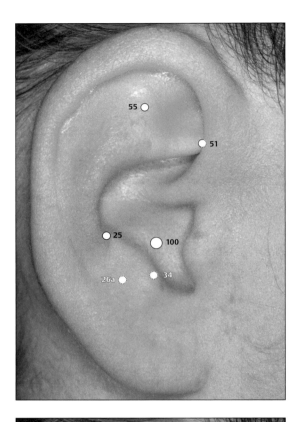

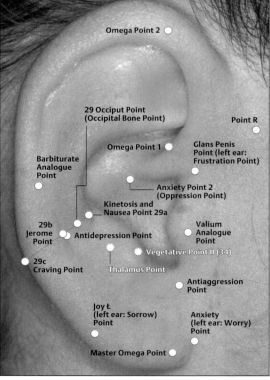

Explanations of the Points Used

Points According to Chinese Nomenclature

25 Brain Stem Point

Location: At the intersection of the antitragus and the anthelix, slightly nearer the antitragus.

Indication: Meningeal irritations, child development problems, consequences of concussion.

26a Pituitary Gland Point
(Thalamus Point According to *Nogier*)

Location: Corresponds on the inside to the location of Point 35 (Sun Point), in the middle of the base of the antitragus.

Indication: A general analgesic point.

▶ According to *Nogier*, affecting the homolateral side of the body.

▶ Caution: Contraindicated during pregnancy.

Occiput Point (Occipital Bone Point According to *Nogier*)

Location: On the outside of the antitragus, below the postantitragal fossa.

▶ *Nogier* locates the Occiput Point in the postantitragal fossa, in the center between Point 29a and Point 29b.

Indication: An important point with a broad spectrum of activity. Conditions of pain, skin diseases, functional circulatory disorders, allergies, vertigo, autonomic dysfunction, phase of recovery.

Gray Substance Point
(Vegetative Point II According to *Nogier*)

Location: On the inside of the antitragus, above the Ovary Point (23 [Eye of the Snake]).

Indication: The point has a general harmonizing effect, antiphlogistic and analgesic activity.

51 Vegetative Point

Location: At the intersection of the inferior anthelical crus and the helix.

Indication: An important point; vegetative stabilization of all visceral organs.

55 *Shen men* ("Divine Gate Point")

Location: In the angle formed by the superior and inferior anthelical crura, more toward the superior anthelical crus.

Indication: An important point. Very effective for emotional stabilization, a point of overriding importance in conditions of pain, anti-inflammatory activity.

100 Heart Zone

Location: In the middle of the inferior concha.

Indication: Psychovegetative dysregulation, hypertension, hypotension, insomnia, anxiety, heart trouble, depression.

Points According to *Nogier* and *Bahr*

29 Occiput Point (Occipital Bone Point)

Location: In the postantitragal fossa, roughly midway between Point 29a and Point 29b. According to Chinese nomenclature, the localization of the Occiput Point is slightly more toward the face.

Indication: An important analgesic point with a broad spectrum of activity. Conditions of pain, skin diseases, functional circulatory disorders, allergies, vertigo, autonomic dysfunction, phase of recovery.

29a Kinetosis and Nausea Point

Location: Between Point 25 (Brain Stem Point) and Point 29 (Occiput Point).

Indication: Kinetosis, vomiting.

29b Jerome Point, Relaxation Point

Location: In the postantitragal fossa, at the intersection with the Vegetative Groove.

Indication: For vegetative harmonization. Difficulty falling asleep. In case of difficulty staying asleep, the corresponding point on the back of the ear is needled.

29c Craving Point

Location: At the end of the postantitragal fossa, at the intersection with the edge of the ear.

Indication: Used as part of addiction therapy.

Antiaggression Point

Location: At the lower edge of the intertragic notch, toward the face.

Indication: An important psychotropic point: addiction treatment (a silver point on the dominant ear).

Anxiety/Worry Point

Location: On the front edge of the lobule at the point where it emerges.

Indication: Anxiety, worry.
In case of right-handedness:

► Anxiety: Treatment via the right ear (silver needle);
► Worry: Treatment via the left ear (silver needle).

In case of left-handedness: vice versa.

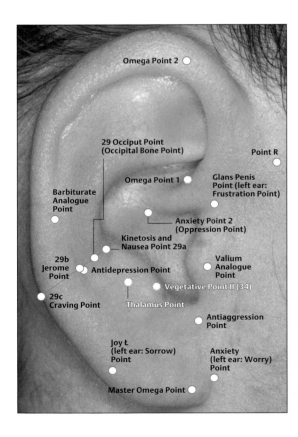

Omega Point 1, Hypogastric Plexus Point

Location: On the upper edge of the crus of helix, toward the superior concha, roughly in the middle between Point Zero and the intersection of the ascending helix and inferior anthelical crus.

Indication: Gastrointestinal and urogenital complaints, renal colic, passing of stones (in addition, Thalamus and Jerome Point).
Bahr: Reference point for amalgam exposure (treatment of dominant ear with gold needle).

Omega Point 2

Location: On the upper edge of the helix, nasal to the Allergy Point 78.

Indication: A point of overriding importance for the motor system.

Master Omega Point

Location: On the lower part of the lobule toward the face.

Indication: An important psychotropic point; intensely effective, harmonizes the vegetative system.

Antidepression Point

Location: On the elongation of the Vegetative Groove, on a line which runs through Point Zero and C1.

Indication: Depressive mood, psychosomatic disturbances.

Valium Analogue Point

Location: On the tragus, roughly 2 mm before the edge of the tragus and just below the middle of the tragus (gold point on non-dominant ear).

Indication: Addiction treatment. The point has general sedating activity.

Vegetative Point II

Location: On the inside of the antitragus, on the caudal leg.

Indication: Analgesic, vegetative harmonization.

Thalamus Point
(26a Pituitary Gland Point According to Chinese Nomenclature)

Location: On the inside of the antitragus, opposite the Temporal Bone Point (Point 35, Sun Point).

Indication: Vegetative harmonization, a general analgesic point, premature ejaculation, frigidity, affecting the homolateral side of the body.

▶ In case of articular rheumatism: use gold needles.

▶ Caution: Contraindicated during pregnancy.

Barbiturate Analogue Point

Location: Half-covered inside the reflex location of the sympathetic medullar original area, in the groove of the ascending helix, at the level of C7.

Indication: Effects similar to barbiturates.

Frustration Point
(Right Ear: Glans Penis Point)

Location: Toward the face on the cranial part of the supratragic notch.

Indication: Frustration, psychosomatic disorders.

Point R (According to *R.J. Bourdiol*)

Location: Elongation of the ascending helix branch, in the fossula at the transition to the face.

Indication: An adjuvant point in psychotherapy.

Eye Diseases

Points According to Chinese Nomenclature

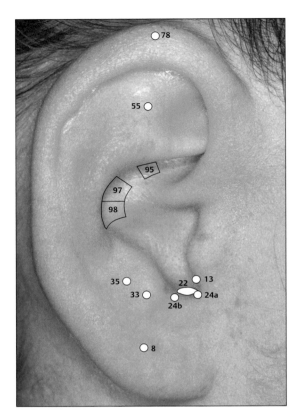

8	Eye Point
13	Adrenal Gland Point
22	Endocrine Point
24a	Eye Point 1
24b	Eye Point 2
33	Forehead Point
35	Sun Point
55	*Shen men*
78	Apex of Ear Point (*Nogier*: Allergy Point)
95	Kidney Zone
97	Liver Zone
98	Spleen Zone

► The indication of Point 24a and Point 24b is specified for all non-inflammatory diseases of the eye. In China diseases such as myopia, astigmatism, and opticus atrophy are treated via these points.

► According to the traditional Chinese school, the liver is linked to the eye (cf. Five Elements). Thus, Point 97 (Liver Zone) is often needled as well in the case of non-inflammatory eye diseases.

Points According to *Nogier*

ACTH Point
Irritated Vertebral Segment Point
Sensory Line (connecting line between Point 29, Occiput Point—Point 35, Sun Point—Point 33, Forehead Point; results in energetic flow through the head).
Allergy Point (78 [Apex of Ear Point] according to Chinese nomenclature)
Eye Point

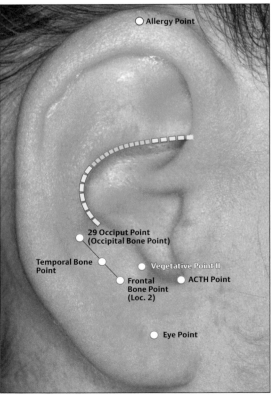

Frequently Found Point Combinations in Eye Diseases

Hordeolum

8   Eye Point
97 Liver Zone
98 Spleen Zone

Conjunctivitis

8   Eye Point
12 Apex of Tragus Point
97 Liver Zone
....
Allergy Point

Glaucoma

8   Eye Point
13 Adrenal Gland Point
29 Occiput Point
35 Sun Point
97 Liver Zone

Macula Degeneration

24a Eye Point 1
24b Eye Point 2
55 *Shen men*
95 Kidney Zone
97 Liver Zone
....
ACTH Point
Points of the Sensory Line (Point 29, Occiput
Point—Point 35, Sun Point—Point 33, Forehead
Point)

▶ Here combination with other somatopes has
proved worthwhile, e.g. oral acupuncture
and new pain and organ treatment via
points. Diagnosis of the field of disturbance
plays an important part.

Dizziness and Tinnitus

Points According to Chinese Nomenclature

- 9 Inner Ear Point
- 22 Endocrine Point
- 34 Gray Substance Point
- 51 Vegetative Point
- 55 *Shen men*
- 95 Kidney Zone
- 96 Pancreas and Gallbladder Zone
- 97 Liver Zone
- 98 Spleen Zone

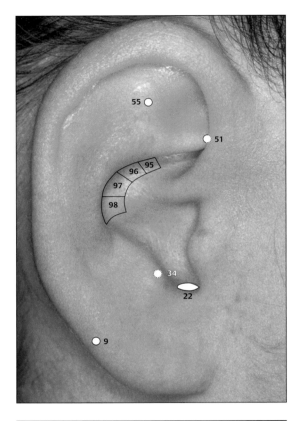

Points According to *Nogier* and *Bahr*

Irritated Vertebral Segment Point

29 Occiput Point

29a Kinetosis and Nausea Point

Temporomandibular Joint Point

Stellate Ganglion Point

Statoacoustic Nerve Zone

Valium Analogue Point

Points of the Sensory Line (Point 29, Occiput Point—Point 35, Sun Point—Point 33, Forehead Point)

Points on the Vertigo Line according to *von Steinburg*

Vertigo Point

- ► The Vertigo Line according to *von Steinburg* is the horizontal line which runs from Point 25 (cf. p. 54) along the upper edge of the antitragus. It is located slightly more to the inside.

- ► The vertical line runs along the postantitragal fossa to the helical groove in accordance with the line of Points 29a, 29, and 29b.

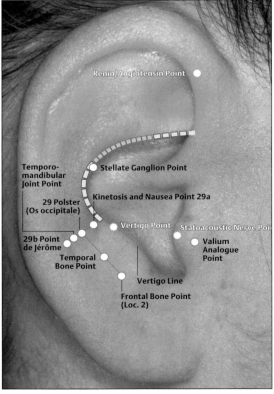

Frequently Found Point Combinations in Conditions of Vertigo and Tinnitus

Tinnitus

9 Inner Ear Point
....
29 Occiput Point
29a Kinetosis and Nausea Point
Irritated Cervical Vertebrae Segment Point
Temporomandibular Joint Point
Stellate Ganglion Point
Statoacoustic Nerve Zone
Valium Analogue Point

Vertigo

9   Inner Ear Point
51   Vegetative Point
55   *Shen men*
....
Vertigo Line according to *von Steinburg*
Points of the Sensory Line (Point 29, Occiput
Point—Point 35, Sun Point—Point 33, Forehead
Point)
Irritated Vertebral Segment Point
Temporomandibular Joint Point
Vertigo Point
Stellate Ganglion Point

Neurological Diseases

Points According to Chinese Nomenclature

2	Roof of Mouth Point
3	Floor of Mouth Point
5	Upper Jaw Point
6	Lower Jaw Point
8	Eye Point
9	Inner Ear Point
11	Cheek Zone
13	Adrenal Gland Point
22	Endocrine Point
25	Brain Stem Point
30	Parotid Gland Point
33	Forehead Point
34	Gray Substance Point
35	Sun Point
52	Sciatic Nerve Point
55	*Shen men*
84	Mouth Zone
87	Stomach Zone
98	Spleen Zone
100	Heart Zone
101	Lung Zone

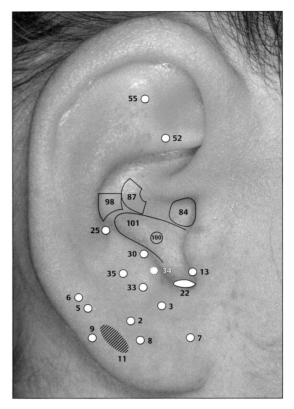

Points According to *Nogier* and *Bahr*

Trigeminal Zone
Point Zero
Weather Point
Irritated Vertebral Segment Point
Valium Analogue Point
Vegetative Point II
Stellate Ganglion Point
First Rib Point
Temporomandibular Joint Point
Barbiturate Analogue Point
Thalamus Point

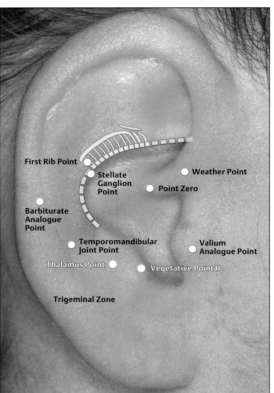

Frequently Found Point Combinations in Neurological Diseases

Trigeminal Neuralgia

5 Upper Jaw Point
6 Lower Jaw Point
8 Eye Point
9 Inner Ear Point
11 Cheek Zone
29 Occiput Point
33 Forehead Point
34 Gray Substance Point
35 Sun Point
....
Trigeminal Zone
Point Zero
Weather Point
Irritated Cervical Vertebrae Segment Point
Temporomandibular Joint Point
Barbiturate Analogue Point
Valium Analogue Point
Stellate Ganglion Point
First Rib Point

Herpes Zoster

29 Occiput Point
30 Parotid Gland Point (antipruritic effect)
55 *Shen men*
....
Stellate Ganglion Point

Facial Paresis

2 Roof of Mouth Point
3 Floor of Mouth Point
8 Eye Point
11 Cheek Zone
13 Adrenal Gland Point
25 Brain Stem Point
29 Occiput Point
84 Mouth Zone
....
Stellate Ganglion Point
Irritated Vertebral Segment Point
ACTH Point
Temporomandibular Joint Point
Valium Analogue Point

Facial Spasm

5 Upper Jaw Point
6 Lower Jaw Point
11 Cheek Zone
25 Brain Stem Point
34 Gray Substance Point
35 Sun Point
55 *Shen men*
....
Irritated Vertebral Segment Point
Valium Analogue Point
Temporomandibular Joint Point

Intercostal Neuralgia

29 Occiput Point
42 Thorax Point
....
Irritated Vertebral Segment Point

Hyperhidrosis

13 Adrenal Gland Point
22 Endocrine Point
29 Occiput Point
51 Vegetative Point
55 *Shen men*
87 Stomach Zone
98 Spleen Zone
101 Lung Zone

Migraine and Cephalgia

Points According to Chinese Nomenclature

8   Eye Point
22 Endocrine Point
23 Ovary Point
26a Pituitary Gland Point
33 Forehead Point
35 Sun Point
51 Vegetative Point
55 *Shen men*
58 Uterus Point
95 Kidney Zone
100 Heart Zone

Points According to *Nogier* and *Bahr*

Irritated Vertebral Segment Point
Occiput Point
Jerome Point
Points of the Sensory Line (Point 29, Occiput
Point—Point 35, Sun Point—Point 33, Forehead
Point)
Vagina Point
Gestagen Point
Weather Point
Point Zero
Sorrow Point
Joy Point
Antiaggression Point
Gonadotropin Point
Temporomandibular Joint Point
Ovary, Testis, Estrogen Point
Thalamus Point

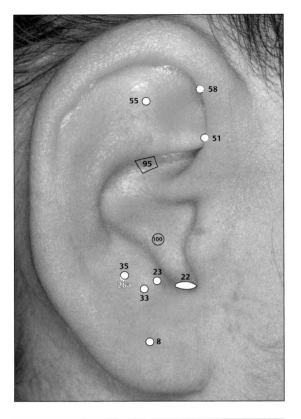

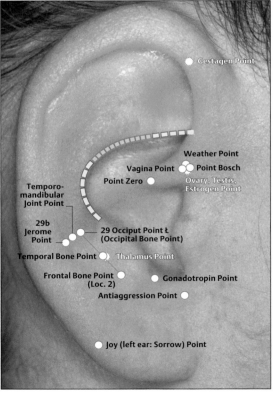

Gynecological Disorders

(K.-H. Junghanns †)

Numerous gynecological disorders upon which drugs have little or no effect can be successfully treated with the aid of acupuncture. In some cases in which a pregnancy only permits the taking of drugs in accordance with strict indications, it is often the only option for responsible treatment. Treatment via the ear has proved particularly advantageous. On the auricula we find not only all the points which are also suitable for acupuncture on the body, but also special points which influence the psyche and hormone production. Proven indications are dysmenorrhea, female sterility for hormonal reasons, and menopausal complaints, above all those accompanied by depressive moods.

During pregnancy, emesis/hyperemesis, imminent abortion, and ischialgia-type complaints may be successfully treated. In hospital it is above all postoperative and postpartum pain, in particular, as well as carcinoma pain, postoperative or postpartum urination problems which respond well to acupuncture.

I. Gerhard and *F. Postneek* from the Gynecological Clinic at the University of Heidelberg, Germany, conducted a study on the treatment of female sterility for hormonal reasons. The greatest successes were with gestagen-positive amenorrhea with normal base hormones and with hyperandrogenemia. The results were comparable with drug treatment but without the unpleasant side effects.

Migraine is a complex disorder which can be triggered by many influences. However, migraine often also has a hormonal component. In uncomplicated migraine, there are no attacks during pregnancy; however, in the case of migraine with aura (flickering before the eyes, impaired sensibility, and vomiting), these attacks also occur during pregnancy. Attention should be paid to this during treatment. Acupuncture treatment is naturally particularly suitable for the treatment of migraine in pregnancy because of the risk attached to taking drugs. In this connection, reference should also be made to the appearance of allergies during pregnancy. Here again, treatment with acupuncture is preferable to treatment with drugs.

Gynecological Disorders

Points According to Chinese Nomenclature

13	Adrenal Gland Point
22	Endocrine Point
23	Ovary Point
51	Vegetative Point
58	Uterus Point
55	*Shen men*
26a	Pituitary Gland Point
52	Sciatic Nerve Point
79	External Genitals Point
95	Kidney, Adrenal Gland Point (functional)
100	Heart Zone

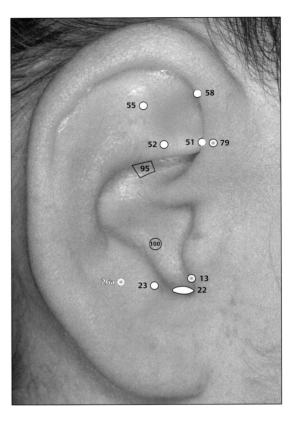

Points According to *Nogier*

Allergy Point

Vegetative Point II

Gestagen Point

Estrogen Point

Gonadotropin Point

ACTH Point

TSH Point

Antiaggression Point

Jerome Point

Valium Analogue Point

Bronchopulmonary Plexus Point

Point R (according to *R.J. Bourdiol*)

Antidepression Point

Laterality Control Point

Thalamus Point

Interferon Point

Thymus Gland Point

Omega Points (1, 2, Master Point)

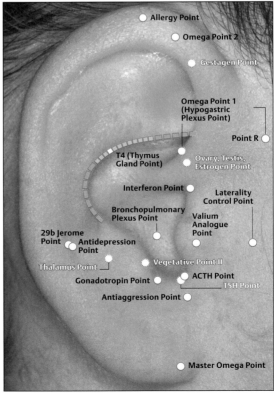

Frequently Found Point Combinations in Gynecology

Dysmenorrhea

55 *Shen men*
58 Uterus Point
....
Gestagen Point
Estrogen Point
Gonadotropin Point

Female Sterility for Hormonal Reasons

Gestagen Point
Estrogen Point
ACTH Point
TSH Point
Gonadotropin Point

Menopausal Syndrome

Gestagen Point
Estrogen Point
Gonadotropin Point

► In cases of aggression, hot flushes, and intermittent sweating and agitation in addition:
Antiaggression Point
Vegetative Points I and II

► In case of insomnia also:
Jerome Point
Valium Analogue Point

► In case of depressive moods also:
Antidepression Point

► In case of laser treatment also:
Bronchopulmonary Plexus Point
Point R (according to *R.J. Bourdiol*)

Ischialgia

55 *Shen men*
52 Sciatica Zone on the side of the complaints
....
Thalamus Point

Emesis/Hyperemesis

Laterality Control Point on both sides

Imminent Abortion

Gestagen Point

Postoperative and Postpartum Pain, Carcinoma Pain

55 *Shen men*
....
Point of the organ concerned
Thalamus Point

Postoperative or Postpartum Urination Problems

Gestagen Point
Estrogen Point
Gonadotropin Point

Allergies during Pregnancy

13 Adrenal Gland Point
78 Allergy Point
....
ACTH Point
Laterality Control Point
Interferon Point
Thymus Gland Point

Urological Diseases

Points According to Chinese Nomenclature

12   Apex of Tragus Point
13   Adrenal Gland Point
22   Endocrine Point
26a Pituitary Gland Point
28   Brain Point
30   Parotid Gland Point
32   Testis Point
51   Vegetative Point
55   *Shen men*
79   External Genitals Point
92   Urinary Bladder Zone
93   Prostate Zone
95   Kidney, Adrenal Gland Point (functional)
100 Heart Zone

Points According to *Nogier*

Testis Point
Prostate Zone
Anus Point
Anxiety Point
Hemorrhoid Point
Omega Points (1, 2, Master Point)
Sorrow/Joy Point
Frustration Point
Hypogastric Plexus Point
Thalamus Point
Jerome Point
Occiput Point

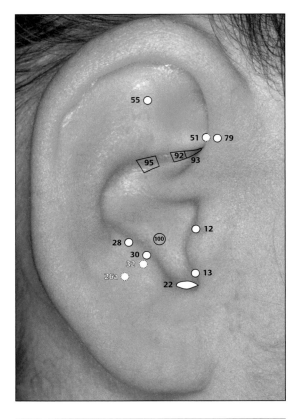

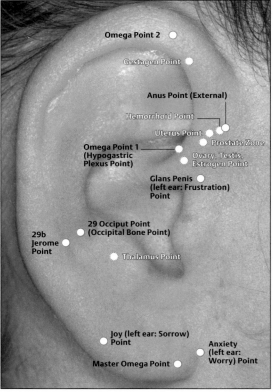

Frequently Found Point Combinations in Urological Diseases

Premature Ejaculation

13 Adrenal Gland Point
22 Endocrine Point
32 Testis Point
79 External Genitals Point
....
Frustration Point
Sorrow Point
Thalamus Point
Jerome Point

Impotence

26a Pituitary Gland Point
28 Brain Point
32 Testis Point
34 Gray Substance Point
95 Kidney Zone
....
Master Omega Point
Thalamus Point

Orchitis

12 Apex of Tragus Point
13 Adrenal Gland Point
32 Testis Point
55 *Shen men*

Prostatitis

12 Apex of Tragus Point
30 Parotid Gland Point
32 Testis Point
92 Urinary Bladder Zone
93 Prostate Zone
....
Jerome Point

Irritated Bladder

29 Occiput Point
30 Parotid Gland Point
51 Vegetative Point
55 *Shen men*
92 Urinary Bladder Zone and Motor
    Bladder Point on the back of the ear
95 Kidney, Adrenal Gland Point (functional)
98 Spleen Zone
....
Kidney Zone
Master Omega Point

Kidney Insufficiency

51 Vegetative Point
95 Kidney, Adrenal Gland Point (functional)
98 Spleen Zone

Kidney Zone

Incontinence

92 Urinary Bladder Zone and Motor
    Bladder Point on the back of the ear
93 Prostate Zone
95 Kidney, Adrenal Gland Point (functional)

Nephrolithiasis

29 Occiput Point
55 *Shen men*
95 Kidney, Adrenal Gland Point (functional)
....
Kidney Zone
Hypogastric Plexus Point

Skin Diseases

Points According to Chinese Nomenclature

13 Adrenal Gland Point
22 Endocrine Point
30 Parotid Gland Point
51 Vegetative Point
55 *Shen men*
71 Urticaria Zone
78 Apex of Ear Point
91 Large Intestine Point
95 Kidney, Adrenal Gland Point (functional)
101 Lung Zone

Points According to *Nogier*

Vegetative Point II
Anxiety Point
Antiaggression Point
ACTH Point
Allergy Point (Chinese Point 78 [Apex of Ear Point])
Occiput Point

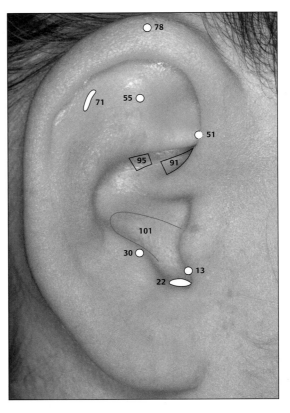

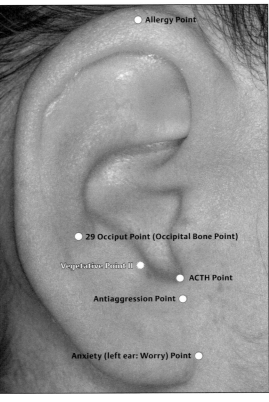

Nervous Control Points of Endocrine Glands

(According to *Bahr*, all the endocrine glands are gold points on the non-dominant ear.)

T12/L1 (Adrenal Gland Point, Loc. 1)
T6 (Adrenal Gland Point, Loc. 2)

Depending on affiliation with one or the other school, different locations are indicated.

Location: Zone III, Adrenal Cortex Point, Cortisone Point.

Indication: Rheumatism, allergies. This point has general anti-inflammatory and analgesic activities.

T12 (Pancreas Point, Loc. 1)
T6 (Pancreas Point, Loc. 2)

Depending on affiliation with one or the other school, different representation zones are indicated.

Location: Zone III, Pancreas Point, Insulin Point.

Indication: Indigestion.

T4 (Thymus Gland Point, Loc. 1)
T1/T2 (Thymus Gland Point, Loc. 2)

Depending on affiliation with one or the other school, different representation zones are indicated.

Location: Zone III, Thymus Gland Point.

Indication: Allergic disorders, counteracts fields of disturbance.

T5 (Mammary Gland Point)

(Also partially indicated as a non-endocrine gland in this area [variation according to school]).

Location: Zone III, Mammary Gland Point.

Indication: Difficulties with breast-feeding, premenstrual mastodynia.

C6/C7 (Thyroid Gland Point)

Location: Zone III, Thyroid Gland Point.

Indication: Thyroid disorders, globus sensation.

C5/C6 (Parathyroid Gland Point)

Location: Zone III, Parathyroid Gland Point.

Indication: Bone diseases, osteoporosis, fracture healing, cramps.

Diseases of the Locomotor System

Projection Zones of the Bony Skeleton According to *Nogier*

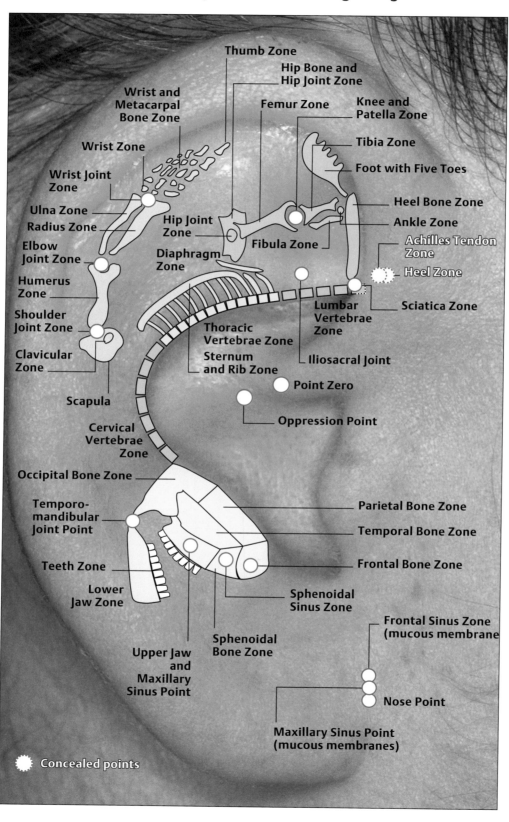

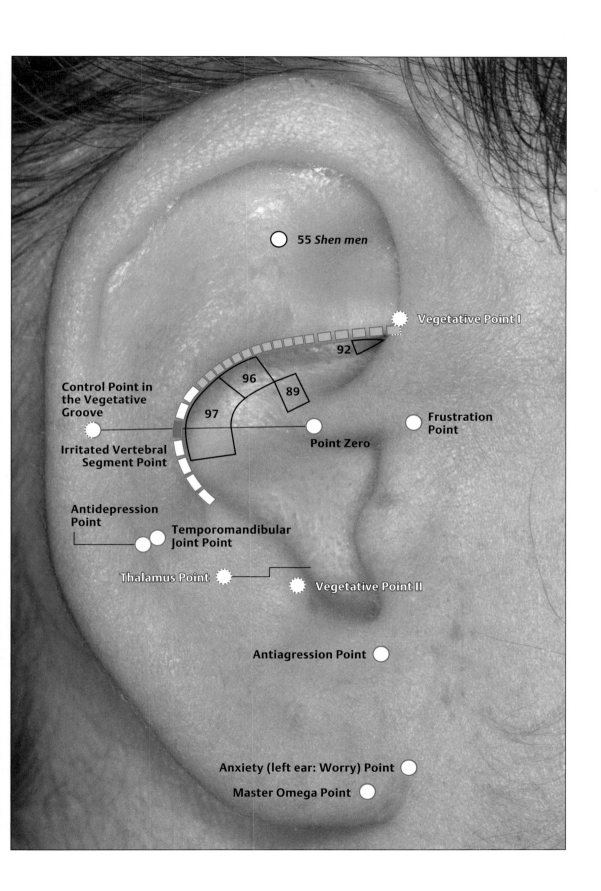

Cervicocephalgia

In clinical terms, headaches in the dorsal region of the head which are experienced as a dull dragging sensation, rarely as a stabbing pain, are to the fore. Vegetative disturbances such as vertigo, slight nausea without vomiting, and tinnitus, which is governed by cervical vertebral column movements, are often encountered.

Acute Disturbances

Acute disturbances are treated with auricular geometry according to *Nogier* supplemented by the Occipital Bone Point (= 29 Occiput Point) and *shen men* (55), possibly also by points with a harmonizing effect on the vegetative system (cf. also p. 159).

Chronic Disturbances

In the case of chronic disturbances, in addition to auricular geometry, superordinate points of the conchae according to TCM are also included. In body acupuncture, as a longitudinal permeation of the head, points BL-2, BL-10, and BL-60 or BL-62 in addition to SI-3 and GV-14 are considered for pain in the region of the Small Intestine/Bladder (*tai yang* axis). In the case of pain in the radial area of the *shao yang* axis (Gallbladder/Triple Burner), TB- 5, TB-15, GB-20, and GB-41 are frequently needled (cf. also p. 166).

Where there are indications that the temporomandibular joint is involved, this should also be included in the treatment. However, in addition to orthopedic functional therapy to eliminate faulty statics of the axis organ, in this case dental treatment must also be provided as well as, for example, in the case of bruxism, the application of relaxation techniques (autogenic training, progressive muscle relaxation according to *Jacobson*).

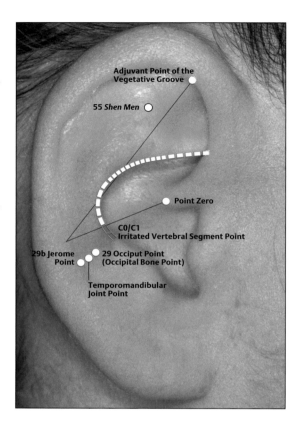

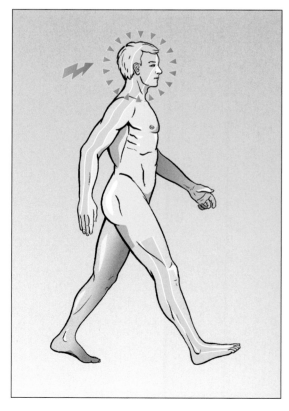

Local Cervical Syndrome

The complaints are purely local and appear for the most part as circumscribed muscular lumps with one-sided restriction of movement. The causes of these are segmental, reversible, functional disturbances of vertebrae which quickly respond to acupuncture.

Acute Disturbances

In the case of acute disturbances, as a rule a combination of auricular geometry according to *Nogier* with *shen men* (55) or the Thalamus Point (26a) are sufficient for more severe complaints. Acute torticollis or acute hyperextension injury is a special case in which manual therapy, which would otherwise be indicated, is no longer or not yet indicated. Here the Jerome Point is used in addition because of its muscle-relaxant effect. With cervical spine distortion, treatment of the Kidney Zone (95) is useful for treatment of the psychosomatic component (fright) at the same time. Other psychotropic points are also used depending on responsiveness.

Chronic Disturbances

Chronic disturbances appear less often as circumscribed local cervical syndrome; combinations with cervicocephalgia and cervicobrachialgia occur on a regular basis. Usually a general static/structural problem or a depressive syndrome is the underlying reason for such a disturbance. Here, in addition to auricular and body acupuncture, an indepth investigation of the causes is indicated, in particular where there is a tendency for the complaints to relapse.

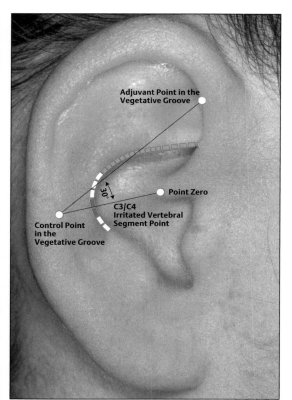

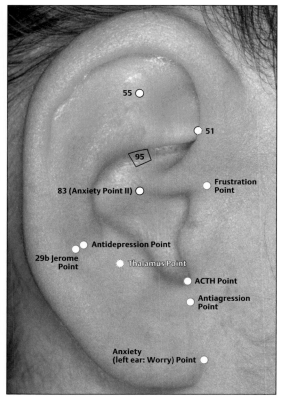

Diseases of the Locomotor System

Cervicobrachial Syndrome

Pain projections in the arm characterize these diseases. Usually they are based on relayed pain in non-radicular incidents so that they respond well to acupuncture. In radicular incidents involving the motor system, the otherwise little used back of the auricula with its representation zones of the motor system may be included. Here too, the distinction between acute and chronic disturbance is useful.

Acute Disturbances

In acute disturbances, auricular geometry is primarily used in the affected area and the concept supplemented according to concomitant modalities.

As obstructions of the first or second rib frequently occur at the same time, even in the case of acute disturbances sensitivity should be detected specifically in the representation zone, as this is a cause of relapse and should therefore be included in the treatment concept at an early stage.

Chronic Disturbances

Chronic disturbances are needled incorporating auricular geometry by means of the needling of superordinate points usually in combination with body acupuncture. When searching for sensitive vertebral motor segments, quite often these are found on several levels; here the most sensitive segment is then treated first and at the next session the sensitivities are tested again before needling.

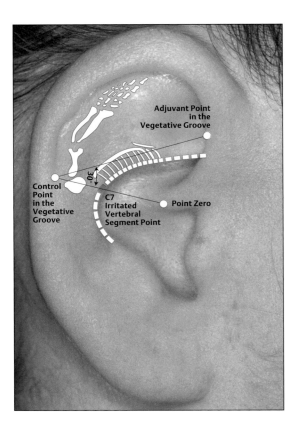

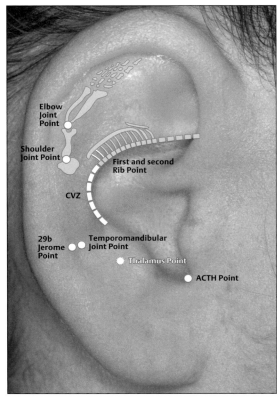

Afflictions of the Upper Extremities

The treatment principle applicable here is as follows: in the case of acute illness, as a rule a local disturbance of the joint concerned may be assumed so that treatment of the joint takes precedence.

On the other hand, in the case of chronic disturbances, there are regularly irritations of proximal or distal joints and the vertebral segment assigned to the affected joint. Distinction from the cervicobrachial syndrome is no longer reliable and is determined by the stage of the disease at which the patient is presented to the acupuncturist.

Diseases of the Locomotor System

Shoulder Joint Disturbances

These subsume diseases which range from purely functional to major structural changes and are roughly summarized under scapulohumeral periarthritis. A simple subacromial bursitis after unaccustomed physical strain can understandably be treated more successfully than a chronic impingement syndrome caused by a rotator cuff rupture. In this respect, in treating diseases of the shoulder girdle, an orthodox medical diagnosis is imperative in assessing the prospect of success of the planned acupuncture.

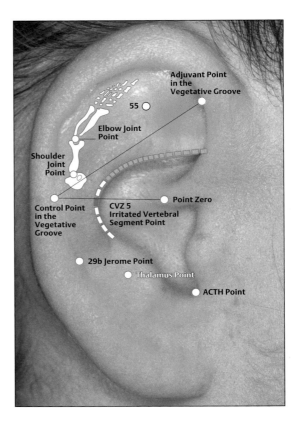

Acute Disturbances

In the case of acute disturbances, treatment is via the shoulder representation zone according to *Nogier*, supplemented by *shen men* (55) with its anti-inflammatory activity and the Jerome Point (29b) with its muscle-relaxant activity. In severe conditions of pain, the Thalamus Point is used. According to the localization of the pain, a distinction is drawn between a ventral, lateral, and dorsal shoulder pain.

Ventral shoulder pain is assignable to the *yang ming* axis (LI–ST) or *tai yin* axis (LU–SP) and is treated via the reflex zones of the large intestine (90) and stomach (87) or lung (101) and of the pancreas/gallbladder (96). Clinical findings and the respective sensitivity of the reflex zones are crucial in the selection of points.

In the axial diagram, lateral shoulder pain corresponds to the *shao yang* axis (TB–GB) and includes the Gallbladder Zone (96); the reflex zone of the Triple Burner (104) usually displays little responsiveness and is therefore seldom needled.

In the case of dorsal shoulder pain, the sensitivity of the Small Intestine Zone (89) and Bladder Zone (92) is tested and if appropriate, needled in accordance with the *tai yang* (SI–BL) axial diagram.

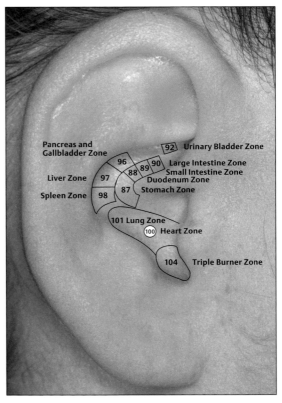

Chronic Disturbances

Besides consideration of the treatment diagrams of acute shoulder pain, the treatment of chronic shoulder pain also requires the inclusion of auricular geometry via the frequently irritated C5 segment and body acupuncture with local and remote points. Likewise, points of emotional stabilization are also taken into consideration.

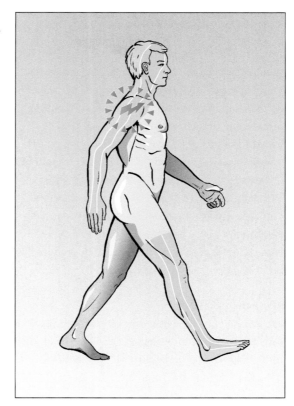

Pain loc.	Dorsal	Lateral	Ventral	Internal
Affected axis	SI–BL *Tai yang*	TB–GB *Shao yang*	LI–ST *Yang ming*	LU–SP *Tai yin*
Ear Points	89 Small Intestine Zone 92 Urinary Blad der Zone	96 Gallbladder Zone 104 Triple Burner Zone	90 Large Intestine Zone 87 Stomach Zone	101 Lung Zone 98 Spleen Zone

Elbow Joint Disturbances

Localization of the complaints is both medial ("pitcher's elbow") and lateral ("tennis elbow"). They are usually acute after unaccustomed use of the muscle group in the vicinity of the elbow joint. Via a muscular imbalance, this often leads via a chronic insertion tendopathy to a disturbance of muscle function chains and functional disturbances of joints. A typical example is pain on the lateral humerial epicondyle, which in the event of its becoming chronic, results in functional disturbances in the C6 segment, the acromioclavicular joint, the proximal radioulnar joint, the scaphoid, and the thumb carpometarpal joint, and therefore leads to resistance to treatment if acupuncture is restricted to purely local treatment.

Acute Disturbances

In the case of acute disturbances, treatment is first restricted to the representation zone of the elbow in the scapha and, depending on localization of the pain, may include the Large Intestine Zone (90) laterally or the Small Intestine Zone (89) medially. In the case of complaints governed by movement, the eminentia scaphae on the back of the ear should also be examined for sensitivities. Further selection of points is based on the concomitant modalities of the acute disturbance: inflammation (ACTH Point), pain (*shen men*, 55), muscle tension (Jerome Point, 29b).

Chronic Disturbances

In the treatment of chronic disturbances, besides considerations regarding local needling, those regarding irritation of myofacial function chains should also be included. Therefore, disturbances in the C6 segment (auricular geometry) to the thumb

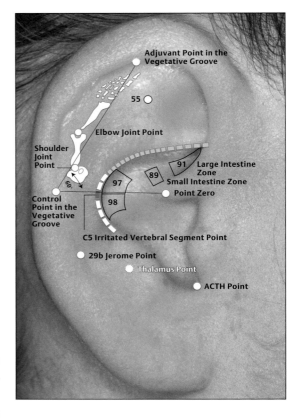

carpometarpal joint play a more significant role than in an acute disturbance.

In combination with body acupuncture, local and remote points corresponding to the axis concerned are included—*shao yin* (HT–KI) in ulnar pain localization, *shao yang* (TB–GB) in dorsal, or *yang ming* (LI–ST) in lateral pain localization.

Yang ming axis	*Shao yang* axis	*Shao yin* axis
90 Large Intestine Zone	96 Gallbladder Zone	100 Heart Zone
87 Stomach Zone	104 Triple Burner Zone	95 Kidney Zone

Hand and Wrist Disorders

Residual complaints after trauma, on the one hand, and degenerative changes, on the other, are chiefly to the fore. However, diseases in the inflammatory–rheumatic group should also be considered. These frequently display polyarthralgia at the prodromal stage without the classic inflammatory characteristics.

Acute Disturbances

In acute disturbances, treatment is via the representation zones of the wrist or the hand in the scapha, including points which reduce inflammation and have an analgesic effect or, if appropriate, also points on the rear side of the ear and, according to the location of the pain, also points on the cavity of concha according to the axial diagram.

Chronic Disturbances

Chronic disturbances necessitate the search for sensitivities of additional reflex zones. Segmental disturbances are found in segments C6 and C7 and T1 and T2.

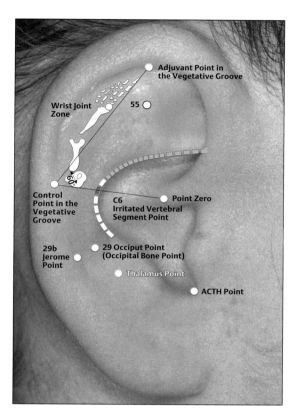

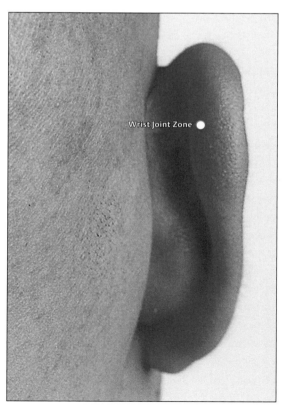

Diseases of the Locomotor System: Spinal Column

Thoracic Outlet Syndrome

Usually this involves the consequences of faulty statics of the spinal column with increased kyphosis or scoliotic deformities. The complaints present as tenseness in overstrained muscle parts. As a rule, obstructions may be found in the irritated vertebral motor segments by means of manual therapy which, on the one hand, include the vertebral joints and, on the other hand, however, the costotransverse joints. These present clinically as pain radiating in the thorax, usually governed by breathing and often permitting the ruling out of a heart attack. Chronic relapse of these complaints is the rule. Therefore, if available, treatment should first be manual/physiotherapeutic/physical, but the use of acupuncture should also be considered.

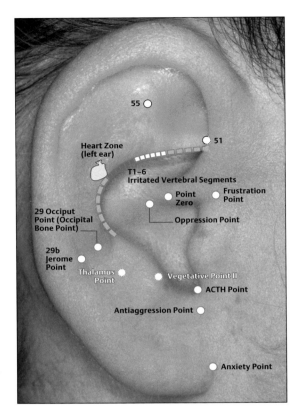

Acute Disturbances

In the case of acute disturbances, in auricular acupuncture the respective, sensitive segments are needled in accordance with auricular geometry according to *Nogier*. Usually both sides of the ears are needled as a purely unilateral, monosegmental disturbance is the exception.

Chronic Disturbances

Chronic disturbances should occasion questions about functional disturbances of organs of the thorax and upper abdomen beyond the limits of orthopedics and, if appropriate, further clarification should be provided. Irritations of segments T1–T3 are associated with those of the lung, segments T4–T6 with those of the heart, the segments below segment T7 with those of the upper abdominal organs. It therefore seems appropriate to also treat responsive areas in the inferior and superior concha in addition to the irritated vertebral segments in auricular acupuncture. With motor disturbances, the back of the ear may also be included in the therapeutic calculation. In spite of careful case history–taking and clinical exploration, cervical spine syndromes are extremely prone to relapse. This is chiefly due to the usually multicausal origin of the complaints which is hard to ascertain down to the last detail and, besides biological factors, also comprises a considerable proportion of psychological factors.

For additional frequently found points, see the illustration.

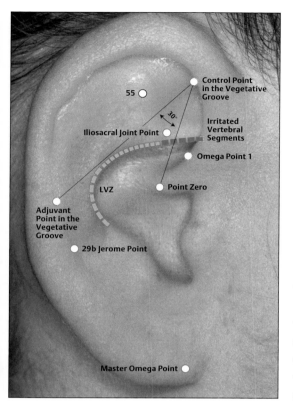

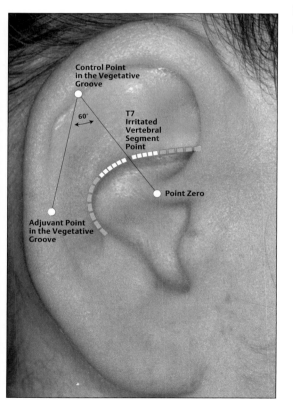

Lumbar Vertebrae–Related Pain Syndrome

Differentiation between a local lumbar spine syndrome and lumboischialgia is made purely for didactic reasons, as in the local lumbar spine syndrome the complaints are usually restricted to the region of the lumbar spine and there is radiating pain in the leg. With lumboischialgia, however, this is frequently the case. All the same, it is usually only at the start of an illness that such a distinction is possible. If this disturbance continues, though, it results in a generalization of pain across the muscle chain with the involvement of several segments, while the origin of this disturbance plays a secondary role in its treatment. Needling is performed according to symptoms and a distinction is not drawn between radicular and nonradicular afflictions as a result of disturbances of the vertebral joints, ligament structures, and musculature. Disease processes outside the vertebral column which have their origin in gastrointestinal, urological, gynecological, or psychosomatic disorders and support a then chronic irritation in the Lumbar Spine Zone should also be included in the differential diagnosis.

Diseases of the Locomotor System

Local Lumbar Vertebrae Syndrome

Often this presents as clinically acute, as a vertebral joint obstruction or lumbago with intradisk mass displacement in the intervertebral disk. Primarily one segment is affected. In auricular acupuncture the clinically identified segment on the representation zone of the inferior anthelical crus is also found to be sensitive on the affected side. Via Point Zero and the affected segment, auricular geometry according to *Nogier* is constructed and sensitive points detected. However, it must be borne in mind that on the other side of the darwinian tubercle the strictly segmental assignment of control points in the Vegetative Groove is no longer specified and in their place, adjuvant points on a second treatment line at an angle of 30°, 60°, 90° in a caudal direction in the Vegetative Groove are usually sought and needled. *Shen men* (55) is used for pain relief and the Thalamus Point (26a) for very severe pain; the Jerome Point (29b) has a muscle-relaxant effect. If there is lumbago, edema responses in the protruding intervertebral disk with accompanying inflammatory response play an important role. Therefore, the ACTH Point, Adrenal Gland Point (13), or Apex of Tragus Point (12) gain in importance here. First, the ipsilateral ear is needled, then, however, the affected segment is also tested contralaterally for sensitivity.

In the process, reduced or increased sensitivity of the ipsilaterally sensitive points is observed. Other vertebral zones may prove responsive instead which, in view of the attack often being multisegmental, is also wholly to be expected. During the course of treatment, the responsiveness of the segmental points and the Thalamus Point declines; instead the psychotropic points (Antiaggression Point, Frustration Point, Anxiety/Worry Point, Sorrow/Joy Point, Antidepression Point) gain in importance. After between five to eight treatment sessions, a significant reduction in complaints is usually to be expected.

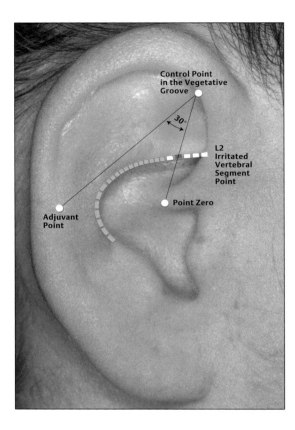

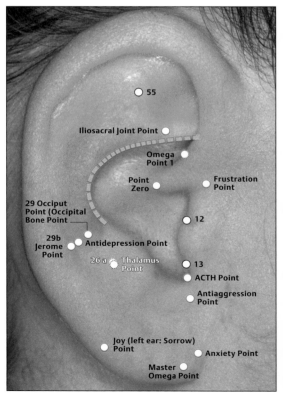

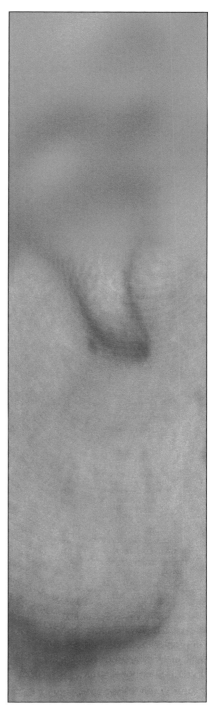

5 The Medical Treatment of Addiction Using Acupuncture

(K. Strauss, J. Blank, K. Spiegel)

The Use of Acupuncture in the Treatment of Drug-Related Diseases
(*K. Strauss, J. Blank*)

Historical Background

Acupuncture treatment for addiction dates back to the early 1970's. In 1972 a neurosurgeon in Hong Kong, Dr. *H.L. Wen*, discovered that opium withdrawal symptoms in a patient had subsided with an ear acupuncture protocol for anesthesia. In the United States, Dr. *Michael O. Smith* and his colleagues, working in the Division of Substance Abuse at Lincoln Hospital, New York, expanded on Dr. *Wen*'s work, and by 1975 had developed what has become known as the NADA 5-point auricular detox protocol (sympathetic, *shen men*, Kidney, Liver, and Heart/Lung).

At that time in the United States, methadone was beginning to be used as a treatment for heroin addiction. Methadone can be taken orally and, due to its considerably longer half-life, once per day dosing is possible. Thus, the complications of i.v. consumption are avoided, making possible an easily administered substitute for heroin. The aim of this substitution is to reduce drug-trafficking crime and to enable addicts to remain fit for work. This method may be useful for some addicts, but it has its drawbacks. Methadone programs are plagued with the problem of "cross-addiction"; in addition to methadone, addicts seek out other drugs, such as alcohol, methamphetamine, marijuana, cocaine, and crack (a cocaine derivative).

In the 1980's, Judge *Herbert Klein* in Miami was given the task of seeking more meaningful ways to give Florida's many crack addicts appropriate treatment. He sought a way for drug addicts to be able to withdraw from opiates as well as cocaine and to reduce their propensity to aggression during the consumption phase if possible. Cocaine has a destructive effect on the psyche. Its aftereffects—psychotic-like episodes—can persist for years and appear completely unexpectedly. There is no substitute for cocaine (as methadone is a substitute for heroin).

This was the situation when *Michael Smith* and Judge *Klein* met. At the time, *Smith* was running the outpatient department for drug addicts at Lin-coln Hospital in New York. He had been working there for years in a program based on the NADA 5-point auricular protocol. The success of the acupuncture-based program at Lincoln convinced Judge *Klein*. Projects supported by the judicial system were started in Florida, as well as several other states, with considerable success.

In 1996, approximately 250 drug addicts a day were treated on an outpatient basis at Lincoln Hospital in New York (chiefly) with auricular acupuncture. The success of this program (i.e. among other things reduced aggression and extension of clean times) was significantly greater than that of other drug withdrawal programs not only in New York but also in other parts of the United States.

However, acupuncture treatment of drug addicts in that country would probably still be eking out its previous wallflower existence today were it not for another—sometimes more important—aspect besides patient success: it is cheaper than other therapies. Nevertheless, astonishingly this form of treatment has only slowly found its way to Europe.

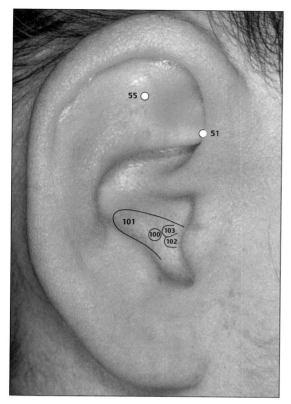

► **102 Bronchial Zone:** medial to the Lung Zone toward the external meatus acusticus.

► **103 Trachea Zone:** above zone 102.

According to *Nogier*, the following auricular points can be included in the treatment plan:

► **Antiaggression Point:** at the lower edge of the intertragic notch, toward the face.

► **Craving Point:** at the end of the postantitragal fossa, at the intersection with the helix.

► **Larynx/Pharynx Point:** upper part of the supra-tragic notch.

► **Occiput Point:** in the postantitragal fossa, roughly midway between points 29a and 29b.

► **Frustration Point:** in the furrow between the tragus and helical crus.

When needling, the most sensitive points are selected each time.

As a rule, treatment takes place every two days in the first week, thereafter once or twice a week depending on requirements, with each treatment lasting 30 minutes.

Treatment usually lasts three to four weeks. Each patient must be individually examined and temporary eating disorders, for example, must be included in the treatment plan.

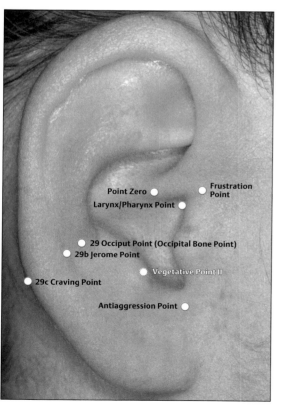

Acupuncture for Obesity

Origin of Obesity According to Traditional Chinese Viewpoints

Obesity should be understood as a multifactorial false regulation of the body, in which both hereditary and genetic factors as well as endocrinological, psychological, and social causes play a role.

Overweight resulting from an increased craving for food responds significantly better to addiction treatment with acupuncture than overweight for hormonal reasons.

According to traditional Chinese viewpoints, weaknesses of individual organ systems, in particular, the Spleen Channel, result in excessive hunger. Weakness of the spleen *qi* can also present as exhaustion, fatigue, weakness, and digestive disorders with bloating and swelling of the extremities.

The patient's tongue is pale with a thin, white coating and reveals tooth imprints on the edge of the tongue.

By increasing body tissue, *yin* is strengthened; *yin* obesity represents protection against weight loss and ego reduction.

Body Acupuncture

Treatment of obesity therefore initially consists of strengthening of *yin*, in particular of the Spleen Channel. Moxibustion of the point SP-6 is often recommendable at the start of treatment.

Tonifying body acupuncture then takes place via the following points:

► **GV-20:** relaxation, calming of the *shen*.

► **SP-6:** tonifies the spleen functional circle, eliminates *qi* stagnation, crossing point of the lower three *yin* channels.

► **ST-36:** general tonification, strengthens stomach, spleen, and food *qi* (*gu qi*), stabilizes the mind (*shen*) and emotions.

Possible supplementary points are:

► **LR-13:** master point of the zang organs, *mu* point of the Spleen Channel, removes stagnation of food.

► **BL-20:** *shu* point of the Spleen Channel.

► **SP-3:** *yuan* point, strengthening of the spleen *qi*.

► **CV-12:** *mu* point of the stomach, master point of the *fu* organs, strengthens the spleen and stomach.

► **HT-7:** *yuan* point of the heart, strengthens the circulation and the psyche, regulates in the event of insufficiency of blood as a result of spleen *qi* weakness.

► **PE-6:** *luo* point of the pericardium, regulates the circulation of *qi*, regulates the middle burner.

Auricular Acupuncture

Auricular acupuncture may be used as an alternative treatment or in combination with body acupuncture. *Mukaino* (1981, 1982) showed that there are special points on the ear that reduce appetite. Stimulation of these points resulted in a reduction of the insulin level with an empty stomach and an increase in gastrin secretion.

Auricular acupuncture can both reduce the sensation of hunger and eliminate contractions of the stomach due to hunger (*Poentinen*, 1995).

A proven treatment method is the needling of the following auricular points (Chinese nomenclature):

► **87 Stomach Zone:** around the ascending helix branch.

► **18 Hunger Point:** in the middle between points 13 and 14 on the tragus.

► **17 Thirst Point:** in the middle between points 12 and 14 on the tragus.

► **51 Vegetative Point:** at the intersection of the inferior anthelical crus and the helix.

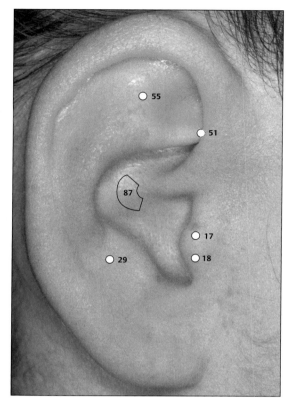

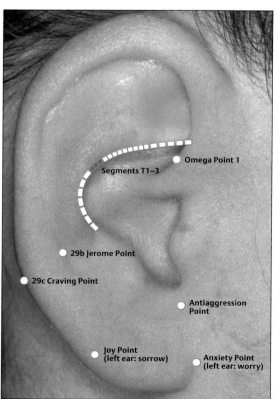

► **55 *Shen men*:** in the angle formed by the superior and inferior anthelical crura, more toward the superior anthelical crus.

According to *Nogier,* the following auricular points can be included in the treatment plan.

► **29 Occiput Point:** in the postantitragal fossa, roughly midway between points 29a and 29b.

► **29b Jerome Point:** in the postantitragal fossa, at the intersection with the Vegetative Groove.

► **Omega Point 1:** in the superior hemiconcha, roughly midway between Point Zero and the intersection of the ascending helix and inferior anthelical crus.

► **Zone of anxiety and worry:** below the Antiaggression Point.

► **Zone of sorrow and joy:** on the occipital part of the lobule, at the same level as the zone of anxiety and worry.

► **Antiaggression Point:** at the lower edge of the intertragic notch, toward the face.

► **Craving Point:** at the end of the postantitragal fossa, at the intersection with the helix.

► **Food Craving Point:** nerval stomach point in zone 2 of the anthelix, affiliated segment T1 to T3.

During needling the most sensitive points are selected each time. Active response zones should always be looked for in the Vegetative Groove.

Treatment takes place once or twice a week and each treatment lasts 30 minutes. It is a long-term treatment and must be geared to the individual.

The Medical Treatment of Addiction Using Acupuncture

Acupuncture In the Treatment of Alcohol Dependency

Symptoms of Alcohol Dependency According to Traditional Chinese Viewpoints

In chronically ill addicts there is usually a *yin* vacuity with a relative excess of *yang*. Patients are anxious and irritable, have night sweating and reddened palms of the hands and soles of the feet. Some have subfebrile temperatures and dryness of the mouth.

An additional kidney *yin* deficiency results in general weakness and lack of strength in the lower back and knee, in part in dizziness, tinnitus, and sexual weakness.

A liver *yin* deficiency is often accompanied by impaired vision, dryness of the eyes, rotatory vertigo, tinnitus, dysesthesia of the extremities, and tremor.

With a heart *yin* deficiency, the patient is often highly mentally excitable, has insomnia and palpitations.

A spleen *qi* weakness results in digestive disorders, edema, muscle weakness, and severe fatigue.

Body Acupuncture

Treatment of alcohol addiction therefore initially consists of strengthening *yin*, as well as, depending on the symptoms, the heart *yin*, the kidney *yin*, the liver *yin*, or the spleen *qi*.

Tonifying body acupuncture then takes place via the following points:

► **SI-20:** relaxation, strengthening of *shen*.

► **HT-7:** *yuan* Point, cooling of heart fire and heart heat.

► **PE-6:** *luo* Point, regulation of *qi*, cooling of heat.

► **GV-14:** calming of *shen*, elimination of heat.

► **KI-3:** strengthening of kidney *yin*.

► **LR-8:** strengthening of liver *yin*.

► **SP-6:** strengthening of spleen *qi*, crossing point of the lower three *yin* channels.

Auricular Acupuncture

Auricular acupuncture may be used as an alternative treatment or in combination with body acupuncture. The following points according to Chinese nomenclature have proved their worth.

► **51 Vegetative Point:** at the intersection of the inferior anthelical crus and the helix. The point may also lie deep in the helical groove.

► **55 *Shen men*:** in the angle formed by the superior and inferior anthelical crura, more toward the superior anthelical crus.

► **97 Liver Zone:** in the middle of the superior semiconcha.

► **100 Heart Zone:** in the middle of the inferior concha.

According to *Nogier*, the following auricular points can be included in the treatment plan.

► **Antiaggression Point:** at the lower edge of the intertragic notch, toward the face.

► **29 Occiput Point:** in the postantitragal fossa, roughly midway between points 29a and 29b. The Chinese localization of the Occiput Point is slightly more toward the face.

► **29c Craving Point:** at the end of the postantitragal fossa, at the intersection with the helix.

► **Vegetative system II:** on the inside of the antitragus, between points 26a (Pituitary Gland Point) and 30 (Parotid Gland Point).

► **Frustration Point:** in the furrow between the tragus and helical crus.

During needling the most sensitive points are selected each time.

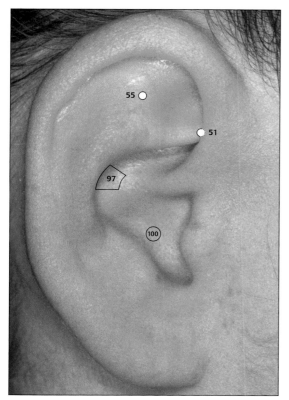

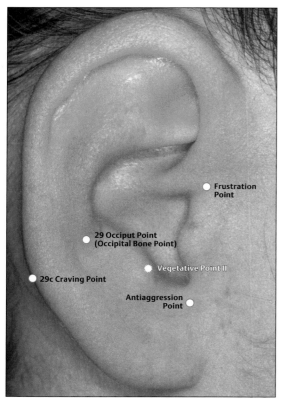

As a rule, treatment takes place daily in the first week, thereafter once or twice a week depending on requirements, with each treatment lasting 30 minutes.

Other Treatment Options

NADA (National Acupuncture Detoxification Association) recommends the following auricular point combination without going into detail about ways of finding the points:

► **Main points:** 51 Vegetative Point, 98 Liver Point, 55 *shen men*, 101 Lung Point, 95 Kidney Point.

► **Additional points:** An additional four points should be selected from the following points according to sensitivity: 97 Spleen Point, 22 Endocrine Point, 29 Occiput Point, 34 Grey Substance Point, 84 Mouth Point, 87 Stomach Point.

Needling is carried out twice a day for 40 minutes each time over a period of four weeks; thereafter once or twice a week for three months.

The Medical Treatment of Addiction Using Acupuncture

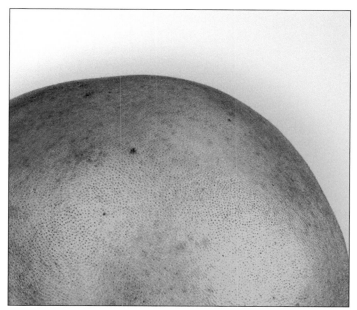

6 Yamamoto New Scalp Acupuncture (YNSA)

(M. Bijak, D. Stockenhuber, H. Nissel)

Presentation of the Method

Around 1970, the Japanese physician Dr. *Toshikatsu Yamamoto* discovered a previously unknown somatope in the region of the head and called it YNSA (Yamamoto New Scalp Acupuncture). Basing his work on the principles of Traditional Chinese Medicine (TCM), he developed a functional, holistic method of diagnosis and therapy that is easy to learn and which in many cases leads to rapid alleviation of complaints.

Implementation

The corresponding points are usually ipsilateral, in other words, located and treated on the side of the body corresponding to the disease. Already during the first treatment with needles, should patients experience at least an improvement in their symptoms. Patients also often report an immediate pain relief as soon as the needle is inserted in the correct place. Depending on the type of disease, the effect remains for a varying length of time. If need be, above all in the case of acute diseases, needling can be performed every day. Further treatment intervals are based on individual circumstances.

In order to ensure the success of the method, as few needles as possible should be used, but these should be placed at exactly the right point.

Every disturbance in the organism is passed on via central mechanisms to the corresponding place in the somatope and there results in a change which is painful for the patient and tangible for the therapist in the sense of a trigger point. When the area concerned is palpated with a finger, a hardened, swollen site is found which is often very painful for the patient. The needle is inserted from caudal to cranial at a slanting angle into as much of this site as possible and left there for approx. 20 minutes.

YNSA may be used alone or in addition to body acupuncture. Taking into consideration the indications and contraindications which correspond to those of traditional acupuncture, no side effects are observed

Subdivision of the Somatope

Anatomically, corresponding to the Structure—Functionally, corresponding to the Condition or Constitution

In principle, an anatomical somatope may be distinguished from a functional somatope. *Yamamoto* calls the zones or points which are assigned to the regions of the body "base points." Base points may be further subdivided into points for the locomotor system and points for the sense organs. For diseases in the region of the brain, the "brain points" are available. If complex disturbances or diseases of "internal organs" are to be treated, the Y-points are another option.

Yin and Yang

Further subdivision takes place through the representation of the zones both on the frontal (*yin*) and on the occipital side of the head (*yang*). These areas are separated by a vertical line that runs through the apex of the ear.

The frontal points are used most frequently for treatment. Only in approx. 2–5% of cases will the occipital points also be necessary for the success of the treatment.

> **Refresher: Fields of application for YNSA points**
>
> ▉ **Frontal and occipital base points:**
> for complaints in the locomotor system.
>
> ▉ **Zones A–I:**
> for diseases of the sense organs (zones for eyes, nose, mouth, ear).
>
> ▉ **Frontal and occipital brain points:**
> for brain diseases.
>
> ▉ **Frontal and occipital Y-points:**
> for complex disturbances.

Division of the scalp into yin *and* yang *areas*

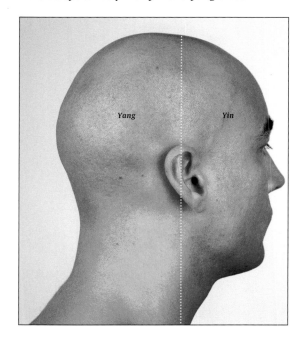

Localization and Indication of the Base Points

Frontal Base Points

These points are effective above all in the case of painful diseases of the locomotor system.

The frontal base points for the locomotor system are located on either side of the median line in the region of the frontal hairline or temple hairline or on the forehead.

Each zone is approx. 0.5 cm wide and 2 cm long. In this area, the trigger zone must first be palpated and then needled. Individual zones are indicated by the letters of the alphabet, with each letter being assigned to a particular region of the body.

Zone A is located 0.5 cm from the median line and stretches from the frontal hairline 1 cm cranial and 1 cm caudal. It is used for the treatment of complaints in the region of the head and the cervical vertebrae. Zone A can be further subdivided in a craniocaudal direction corresponding to the individual cervical vertebrae. The atlanto-occipital joint is the furthest cranial, the cervicothoracic transition caudal.

Zone B runs 0.5 cm lateral and parallel to zone A. It is also used for the treatment of cervical vertebrae and the shoulder girdle. The extension corresponds to Zone A, but there is no further division.

Zone C is described in the region of the "receding hairline." If one imagines a 90° angle which is formed by a horizontal line through the eyebrows and the median line and halve this angle, Zone C is located on this line also starting from the hairline 1 cm cranial and 1 cm caudal. The indications for this zone comprise all disturbances of the upper extremity and the shoulder. According to the anatomy, this zone is also further subdivided with the shoulder projected at the cranial start of the zone, the elbow joint precisely at the hairline, the fingers are located at the caudal end of the zone on the forehead.

Next comes Zone E, which is assigned to the thoracic vertebral column and the thorax. discovered later than Zone D for the lower half of the body. For anatomical reasons, however, it is described before Zone D here.

Zone E is located on the forehead. Starting from the body acupuncture point GB-14 it extends diagonally down in a medial direction to the acupuncture point BL-2. Corresponding to the 12 thoracic segments, this zone is subdivided from cranial to caudal, where T1 is cranial and T12 caudal. The indications comprise not only all functional disturbances of the Thoracic Vertebrae Zone (TVZ) but also diseases in the region of the thorax, such as, for example, intercostal neuralgia or herpes zoster, can be treated via this zone.

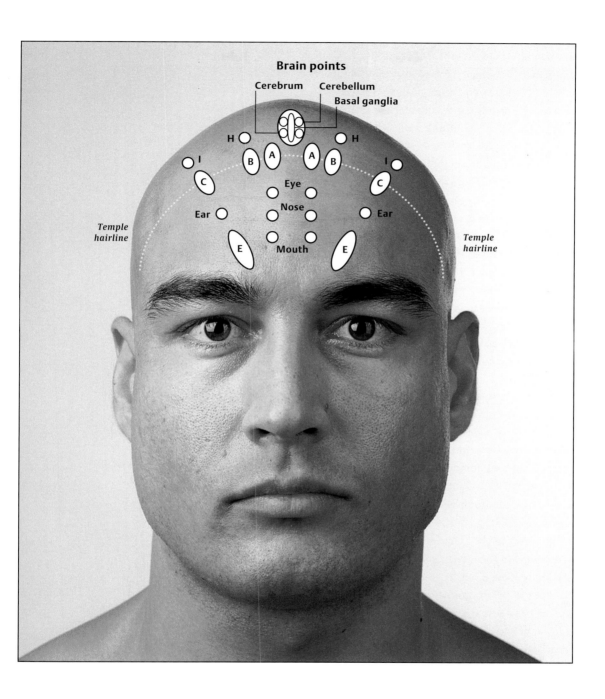

Zone D represents the lower half of the body and is located 0.5–1 cm cranial to the upper edge of the zygomatic arch. It runs from the temple hairline horizontally 1 cm dorsal and 1 cm frontal. Diseases and pain in the region of the lumbar vertebral column and the lower extremity can be treated via this zone, which is not subdivided any further.

Yamamoto cites additional zones not based on the hairline for the treatment of lumbago, ischialgia, and knee and hip complaints.

Another segmented Zone D corresponding to the five lumbar vertebrae located in front of the ear is described. D1–D5 lies vertically just in front of the ear and extends from the base of the upper ear muscle to the upper edge of the zygomatic arch.

All zones of the *yin* side described in the above are also to be found on the *yang* side of the head and are described in brief below. Zones F and G discussed below are actually on the *yang* side, but are nevertheless included in the frontal base points, as no counterpart has yet been found on the *yin* side.

Zone F is retroauricular above the highest point of the mastoid, cranial to the body acupuncture point TB-17. In addition to Zone D, this zone can be treated along the sciatic nerve in the event of radicular or pseudoradicular pain.

Zone G curves around the apex of the mastoid and is divided into three sections. The first section, G1, is ventral to the mastoid apex immediately behind the earlobe and is used for the treatment of complaints in the medial knee joint region. The second section, G2, is located immediately under the apex of the mastoid. Dorsal knee joint complaints can be treated from this point. The lateral knee joint is represented by Zone G3, which is located in the dorsal section of Zone G.

For many years, *Yamamoto* has been searching intensively for further zones of correspondence in this somatope. Just recently these aforementioned zones were thus extended to include regions H and I.

Zone H is cranial next to Zone B; Zone I is next to Zone C. Both zones may be needled in addition to Zone D in the case of hip complaints or lumbago.

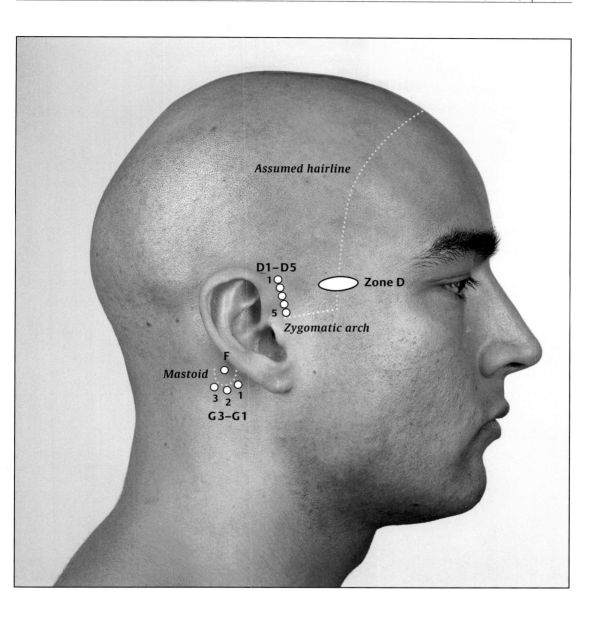

Brain Points

The important "brain points" zone is located on either side of the median line and next to Zone A extending 2 cm in a cranial direction. If the cause of a disease lies in the brain, as for example in all consequences of cerebral insult, treatment can be given via this zone (in addition to or instead of the frontal base points). In these cases, needling is contralateral. The zone itself appears pear-shaped, with the region of the cerebellum in the most dorsal location. The basal ganglia are projected in the area of the median line.

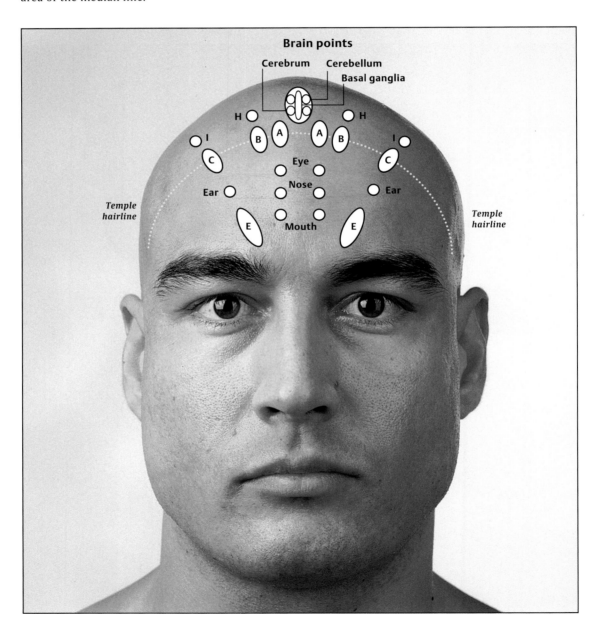

Points for the Sense Organs

The points for the sense organs are located in the area of the forehead and are approx. 1 cm long. Eye, nose, and mouth are located under the other on a vertical line, immediately caudal to Zone A. All functional diseases of these organs are possible indications, such as, for example, conjunctivitis, rhinitis, but also facial paresis, herpes labialis, etc.

The ear is below Zone C on this imaginary line which divides in half the angle between a horizontal line through the eyebrows and the median line. This zone is very often used for tinnitus.

Refresher: Overview of the frontal base points

- **Zone A** ▸ Head, Cervical Vertebrae Zone (CVZ), division C1–C8

- **Zone B** ▸ CVZ, shoulder girdle, undivided

- **Zone C** ▸ Shoulder, upper extremity, division in accordance with anatomy

- **Zone E** ▸ TVZ, thorax, division T1–T12

- **Zone D** ▸ Lumbar Vertebrae Zone (LVZ), lower half of the body, unsegmented

- **Zone D 1–D 5**
  ▸ Corresponding to the 5 lumbar vertebrae

- **Zone F** ▸ Sciatic nerve

- **Zone G** ▸ Knee joint, division G1–G3

- **Zone H and I**
  ▸ Hip, LVZ, used additionally

- **Brainpoints**
  ▸ Head, brain

- **Sense organs**
  ▸ Eyes, nose, mouth, and ear

Occipital Base Points

In approximately 2% of patients, use of the frontal base points alone does not lead to the desired success. In this case, it is also possible to needle the corresponding zones on the occipital side of the head. Very often this treatment will then result in a significant improvement.

With the exception of Zones G and F, the localization of which is only occipital, there is both frontal and occipital projection of all the other zones at the corresponding place. The lambda suture is the counterpart to the forehead or temple hairline here. In contrast to the location of the frontal points, the occipital points are shifted approximately 10° caudal.

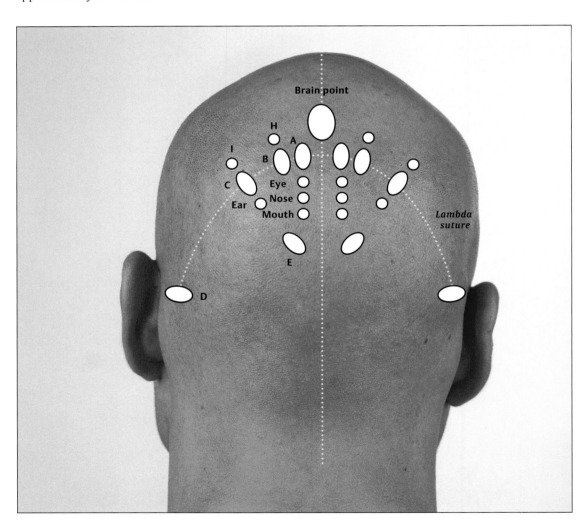

Diagnostic Somatopes

New Abdominal Wall Diagnosis According to *Yamamoto*

In the area of the abdominal wall there are test zones for the 12 channel lines or organs. By palpating these coin- to palm-sized areas, disturbances in the functional circles or organs can be detected. Palpation is initially gentle, with swelling of the subcutis palpable. When the pressure is increased, myogeloses in the area of the abdominal wall can be felt. The patient experiences an "unpleasant feeling" or even pressure pain.

Localization of the Zones of the Abdominal Wall

There are five test areas in the region of the median line, i.e. the Conception Vessel. The Heart Zone is the most cranial, immediately under the Xyphoid. Distal to it is the Pericardium Zone and above the navel, the Stomach Zone.

The **Triple Heater** Zone is immediately below the navel and the **Bladder** Zone above the symphysis. The test areas for **gallbladder** and **spleen** are under the right or left costal arch, according to their anatomical localization. The **Lung** Zone is diagonally right and cranial to the navel. The **Liver** Zone is in the corresponding place on the left. The **large intestine** is projected caudal to the liver and the **small intestine** on the right-hand side at the same level. The **Kidney** Zones, which are the only organ projections arranged in pairs, are localized on the left and right cranial to the inguinal area. A conspicuous palpation finding on one side, however, is sufficient for diagnosis.

Treatment for organs which are conspicuous during palpation, in other words, irritated, is carried out via the Y-points. The abdominal wall is a purely diagnostic somatope. If several test zones prove conspicuous, first the Y-point of the more significant organ according to TCM is needled. If the corresponding Y-point is needled correctly, the abdominal wall finding improves at once.

Test areas for the brain (right brain on the right; left brain on the left) are located on both sides in the angle between Xyphoid apex and costal arch. If there is swelling in this area, treatment is carried out via the brain points already discussed. However, there are also purely anatomical correspondences for the spinal column on the abdominal wall. These extend along the median line from the pericardium zone to the symphysis in accordance with the anatomical location of cranial to caudal of C1 to the coccyx. The thoracic vertebral column arches around the navel. Treatment of diagnosed complaints of the vertebral column is carried out via the corresponding base points.

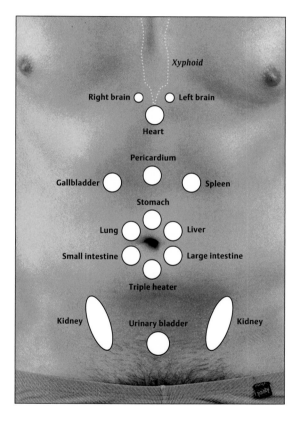

YNSA Neck Diagnosis

The neck triangle, also used exclusively for diagnosis, is located above the clavicle between the front edge of the trapezius muscle and the lateral part of the sternocleidomastoid muscle. A horizontal line through the laryngeal prominence serves as the upper limit.

In this case, as a result of the smaller anatomical proportions, the test areas are rather points. They respond faster and more sensitively, which is an advantage compared with abdominal wall diagnosis.

Irritated organs or functional circles are detected by means of the marked painfulness of the respective points when pressure is applied.

Treatment is carried out via the corresponding Y-points. With correct needling, the sensitivity of the test points in the neck triangle changes at once.

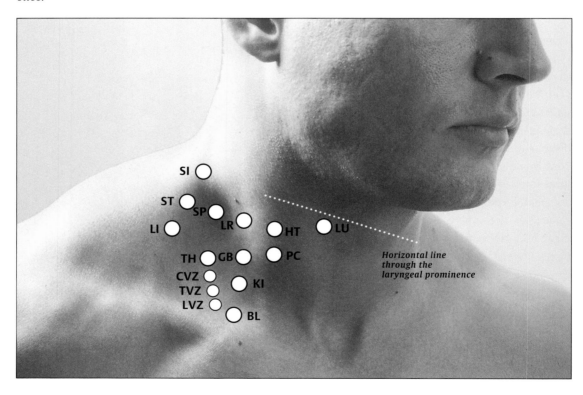

Horizontal line through the laryngeal prominence

Localization of the Zones of the Neck Triangle

The test point for the **bladder** is just above the clavicle in the angle with the dorsal edge of the sternocleidomastoid muscle and that for the **kidney** just above it. The **gallbladder** is localized cranial to it, also on the dorsal edge, and proximal to it the **liver**.

The test point for the **stomach** is located on the front edge of the trapezius muscle, at the level of the lower edge of the thyroid cartilage. Cranial to it is the test point for the **small intestine** and caudal that of the **large intestine**. The **spleen** is projected between the stomach and liver points. The test point for the **triple heater** is caudal to these, roughly between the kidney and large intestine. The points for the **heart** and **pericardium** are directly below a horizontal line through the lower edge of the thyroid cartilage, but on the sternocleidomastoid muscle, i.e. in front of the liver and gallbladder. The **lung** is projected furthest to the front, i.e. on the front edge of the sternocleidomastoid muscle between the horizontal line through the laryngeal prominence and that through the lower edge of the thyroid cartilage.

Besides these test points, there are also purely anatomical test points for the spinal column in the neck triangle. Between the points of the triple heater and the bladder, the **cervical vertebrae** are projected uppermost, diagonally below them the **thoracic vertebrae**, and diagonally below them in turn the **lumbar vertebrae**. These zones only serve to confirm the diagnosis or to monitor treatment. The actual treatment of spinal column complaints is naturally via the base points again.

Y-Points as Functional Somatotope

As already discussed, the base points represent an anatomical somatope. Selection of the zones to be treated takes place according to the localization of the complaints.

On the other hand, the Y-points represent a functional somatope according to TCM. The selection of Y-points takes place—depending on the affected organ or channel line, or following assignment to a particular functional circle—after palpation of the "diagnostic zones" on the abdominal wall or the test points in the area of the neck triangle. They provide the opportunity for constitutional treatment and therefore come in useful in particular for complex disturbances, internal diseases, health disorders, or failure to respond to treatment via the base points or body acupuncture.

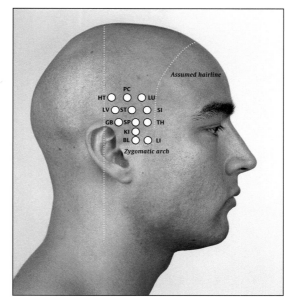

Localization of the Y-Points

The Y-points are projected on the side of the scalp in both the *yin* and *yang* region. As the frontal points are the most important in terms of treatment and the occipital points are of more theoretical interest, only the former will be discussed in more detail here.

The temple hairline, the zygomatic arch, and a vertical line through the apex of the auricle are used as "auxiliary lines" to locate the individual points.

Large intestine: The Y-point of the large intestine lies in the angle formed by the temple hairline and the upper edge of the zygomatic arch.

Urinary bladder: The urinary bladder point is at the same level in the middle of the hairline.

Kidney: The kidney is localized immediately above the bladder.

Gallbladder: The Y-point of the gallbladder lies immediately in front of the point where the upper ear emerges.

Lumbar vertebrae: Zone D1–D5 for the lumbar vertebrae already discussed with regard to base points extends caudal to the gallbladder.

Triple heater: The triple heater is projected at the same level as the gallbladder on the temple hairline.

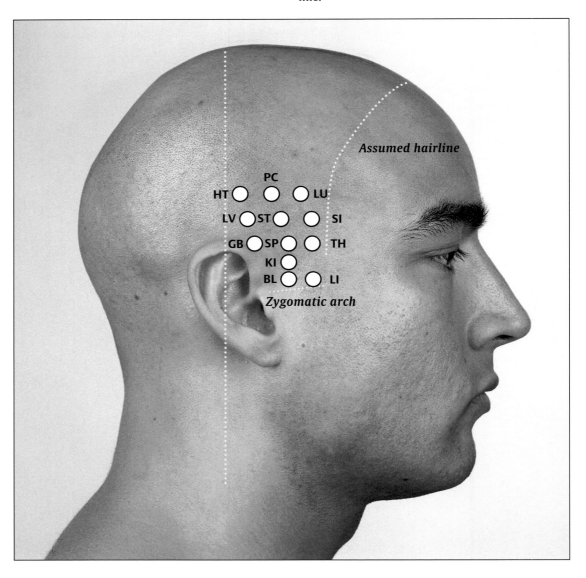

Spleen: Between gallbladder and triple heater.

Liver: The Y-point for the liver is approx. 1 cm above the auricle and a little in front of the vertical line through its highest point.

Stomach: The stomach point is more frontal at the same level as the liver.

Small intestine: That of the small intestine is at the same level as the stomach, but at the hairline.

Heart: The Y-point of the heart is approx. 1 cm cranial to the liver, but closer to the vertical line.

Pericardium: In front of the heart point.

Lung: The lung is projected at the same level as the pericardium, but approx. 1 cm inside the hairline.

The points are found by palpating with the thumb or index finger, as for the base points.

Indications for the Y-Points

In the event of disturbances of the locomotor system and the sense organs, the Y-points may be used in addition to the base points. Equally, they represent an appropriate option for the treatment of diseases of internal organs according to TCM, in other words, for functional, reversible diseases and psychosomatic disorders. It should be pointed out that prior orthodox medical diagnosis is essential in this connection.

Practical Application

In the case of diseases of the internal organs, health disorders, and other functional disturbances, an abdominal wall and/or neck diagnosis is first carried out. This usually indicates the same Y-point as being worthy of treatment. This point is subsequently needled. In diseases which are assigned to one half of the body, the Y-point may be treated together with a corresponding base point on the ipsilateral side. Paralyses of central origin that are treated with acupuncture by means of the brain point on the contralateral side are the exception. If frontal base points are also used, these are usually needled on the ipsilateral side of the pareses.

If a disturbance is not assigned to either half of the body, the side of the body is selected in accordance with whether the patient is right- or left-handed. If needling fails to have the desired effect on that side, the other side is treated.

In the case of frontal Y-points, the needle is inserted from frontal to occipital and at the same time from caudal to cranial into the center of the swelling. Treatment should involve as few needles as possible. In the case of acute indications, short treatment intervals (possibly daily) are recommended; in the case of chronic diseases, treatment is given once a week. The needles are left in for approx. 20 minutes.

The number of treatments required is based on both the chronicity of the disease and the patient's response to treatment.

Yamamoto New Scalp Acupuncture (YNSA)

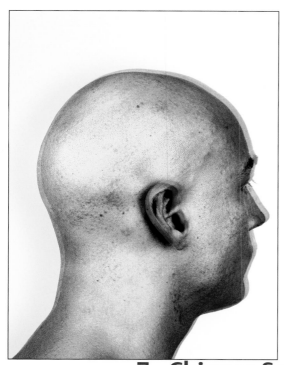

7 Chinese Scalp Acupuncture

(H.-U. Hecker, A. Steveling, E.T. Peuker)

Introduction

Chinese scalp acupuncture is not an actual somatope. The Chinese have rather described certain reflex zones on the scalp from which specific influence can be brought to bear on motor and sensory disturbances.

Fourteen main treatment zones are distinguished:

1. Sensibility Zone
2. Motor Zone
3. Antitremor Zone
4. Vasomotor Zone
5. Vertigo and Auditory Zone
6. Speech Zone II
7. Psychomotor or Associative Zone
8. Sensomotor Zone of the Lower Extremity
9. Speech Zone I
10. Optical Zone
11. Equilibrium Zone
12. Thorax Zone
13. Abdominal Zone
14. Genital zone

In Europe, Chinese scalp acupuncture is very closely associated with the name *Zeitler*.

This late colleague of the Viennese School rendered outstanding services in the development of this method.

Most Important Projection Zones

Sensibility Zone (1)

Location: Connecting line between GB-7 and *du mai* 20 (GV-20). This zone is the most occipital.

Indication: Impaired sensibility, pain. An adjuvant effect in the treatment of phantom limb pain is described. Trigeminal neuralgia, toothache.

Motor Zone (2)

Location: The zone adjoins the Sensibility Zone in the direction of the nose at a distance of 1 cm and runs parallel to this.

Division of the Motor Zone for orientation purposes produces roughly five equal parts:

► The lower extremity, the trunk, as well as the bladder and rectum are located in the area of the upper fifth. As a rule, treatment is contralateral. Where assignment is unclear, acupuncture is performed bilaterally (e.g. bladder).

► The second fifth corresponds to the treatment zone for the upper extremity.

► The hand and finger are represented in the third fifth.

► Trigger points for motor disturbances in the region of the facial musculature are frequently found in the fourth and fifth fifth of the Motor Zone. Swallowing and chewing complaints can also be treated via this projection zone.

Antitremor Zone (3)

Location: The zone adjoins the Motor Zone in the direction of the nose at a distance of 1 cm and runs parallel to this.

Indication: Tremor in the context of Parkinson disease

Vasomotor Zone (4)

Location: In the direction of the nose, furthest to the front and parallel to the Antitremor Zone.

Indication: Adjuvant treatment of hypertension is possible via this zone. Treatment of edema in the case of cerebral pareses is also described.

Vertigo and Auditory Zone (5)

Location: The line is roughly 4 cm long and approx. 2 cm above the apex of the ear.

Indication: Treatment of conditions of vertigo of various origins (vertebrobasilar insufficiency, Ménière disease).

Speech Zone II (6)

Location: Starting from approximately the center of the Vertigo and Auditory Zone in the direction of the occiput, below the Vertigo and Auditory Zone.

Indication: As part of the treatment of sensory aphasia.

Psychomotor or Associative Zone (7)

Location: In the region of the parietal tubercle. The zone is roughly shaped like an isosceles triangle with sides approx. 3 cm long.

Indication: Associative disturbances, ataxia.

1 *Sensibility Zone*
2 *Motor Zone*
3 *Antitremor Zone*
4 *Vasomotor Zone*
5 *Vertigo and Auditory Zone*
6 *Speech Zone II*
7 *Psychomotor or Associative Zone*

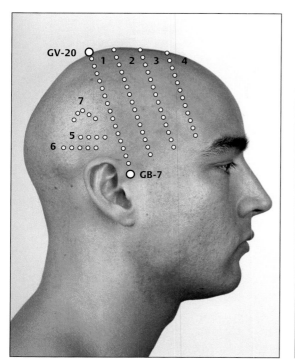

Division of the Motor Zone for orientation

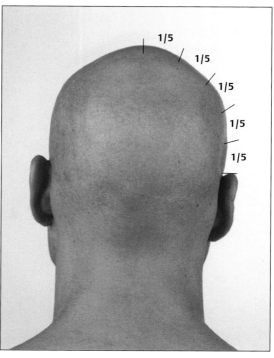

Chinese Scalp Acupuncture

Four further zones may be distinguished in the direction of the occiput.

Sensomotor Zone of the Lower Extremity (8)

Location: Parallel to the median line (connecting line between EX-HN-3 and GV-16). Starting from the center of this line extending approx. 3 cm in the direction of the occiput.

Indication: Sensitive and/or motor disturbances of the lower extremity and as part of the treatment of peripheral edema. Furthermore, infantile enuresis and hysteroptosis are indicated.

Speech Zone I (9)

Location: Approx. 2 cm behind the parietal tubercle, parallel to the median line (connecting line between EX-HN-3 and GV-16).

Indication: Motor aphasia, alexia.

Optical Zone (10)

Location: Approx. 3.5 cm lateral to the exterior occipital protuberance, parallel to the median line (connecting line between EX-HN-3 and GV-16).

Direction: Frontal.

Indication: Chiefly for centrally impaired vision.

Equilibrium Zone (11)

Location: Parallel to the median line, approx. 3.5 cm lateral to the exterior occipital protuberance, caudal.

Indication: Conditions of vertigo the cause of which is related to the cerebellum.

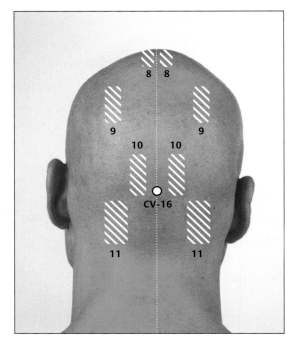

8 Sensomotor Zone of the Lower Extremity
9 Speech Zone I
10 Optical Zone
11 Equilibrium Zone (aid to localization: GV-16, exterior occipital protuberance)
12 Thorax Zone
13 Abdominal Zone
14 Genital Zone

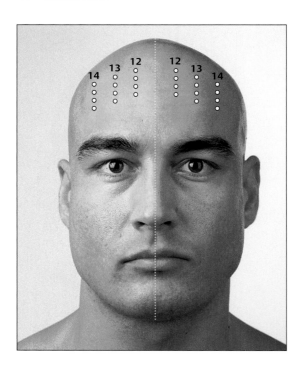

Three zones can be distinguished at the front. They are all in the area of the hairline.

Thorax Zone (12)

Location: In the hairline, above the medial edge of the eyebrow.

Indication: Bronchitis, asthma, dyspnea, pain in the chest.

Abdominal Zone (13)

Location: In the hairline, roughly at the level of the center of the eyebrow.

Indication: Abdominal complaints.

Genital Zone (14)

Location: In the hairline, approx. 2 cm lateral to the Abdominal Zone.

Indication: Genital disorders, abdominal complaints.

Methodology

It goes without saying that the scalp should be examined in detail for any defects before performing acupuncture.

In the treatment of paralyses, we usually find the reflex zones in the region of the scalp zones contralateral to the paralysis. However, examination of both zones is useful, as trigger points occurring on both sides should also be needled on both sides, regardless of the localization of the paralysis. The best results are described using acupuncture up to the scalp periosteum.

To localize the trigger points, the thumb is run over the suspected area exerting a constant pressure. As a rule, in the event of a disturbance the patient then indicates a circumscribed trigger point or a zone which is needled.

With Chinese scalp acupuncture, treatment is carried out at short, one- to two-day intervals.

Of course, this treatment of paralyses only makes sense with additional, effective physiotherapy.

Chinese Scalp Acupuncture

8 Oral Acupuncture

(J. Gleditsch)

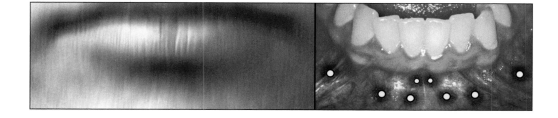

Introduction

Oral Acupuncture is based on a somatotope of reflex points in the oral cavity. The enoral points are situated in the mucous membrane. They were discovered and established in the 1970's, following many years of observation. As an ear, nose and throat specialist as well as a dentist, I carried out my investigations and observations on many thousands of patients. In this way, the concept of Oral Acupuncture emerged.

The oral microsystem has proved to be useful both in diagnosis and therapy. In case of functional disorders of inner organs, specific points in the oral mucous membrane become sensitive to pressure. Owing to the points' increased sensitivity, they can be clearly distinguished from their surroundings. Treatment of such activated points may regulate the dysfunctions of correlated organs and their functions.

Immediate effects are common in Oral Acupuncture, similar to those in auricular and in scalp acupuncture.

In Oral Acupuncture there are five groups of points:

1. **Vestibular points, situated labially and buccally to the adjacent teeth**

2. **Retromolar points, situated beyond the wisdom teeth**

3. **RAM points, situated at the ramus ascendens mandibulae**

4. **Frenular points, situated next to the frenula**

5. **Extraoral points, analogous to the enoral vestibulum points, especially labial points**

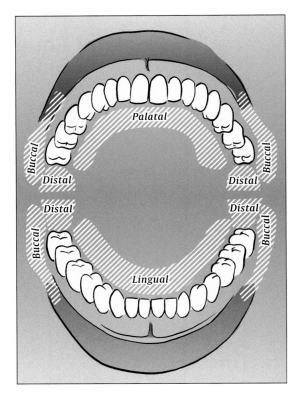

Anatomical areas in the oral cavity

Projection Diagrams of the Retromolar Zones in Quadrants I–II

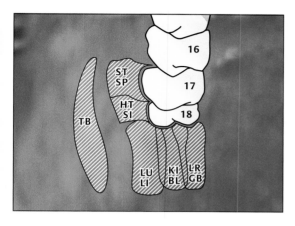

Quadrant I

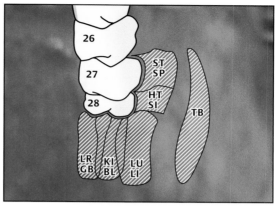

Quadrant II

TB Triple Burner Zone
ST Stomach Zone
SP Spleen Zone
HT Heart Zone
SI Small Intestine Zone
KI Kidney Zone
BL Urinary Bladder Zone
LU Lung Zone
LI Large Intestine Zone
LR Liver Zone
GB Gallbladder Zone

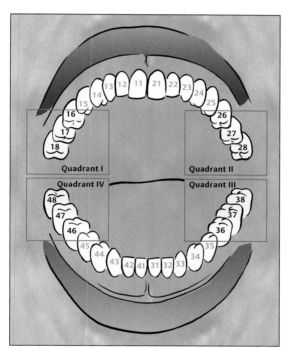

Oral Acupuncture

Projection Diagrams of the Retromolar Zones in Quadrants III–IV

TB Triple Burner Zone
ST Stomach Zone
SP Spleen Zone
HT Heart Zone
SI Small Intestine
   Zone
KI Kidney Zone
BL Urinary Bladder
   Zone
LU Lung Zone
LI Large Intestine
   Zone
LR Liver Zone
GB Gallbladder Zone

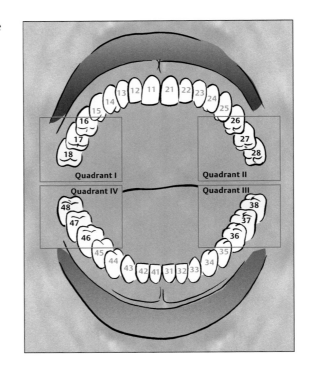

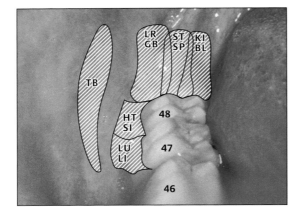

Quadrant III

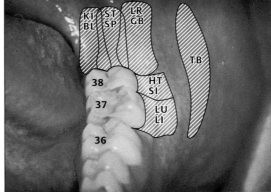

Quadrant IV

Functional Network: Kidney–Bladder

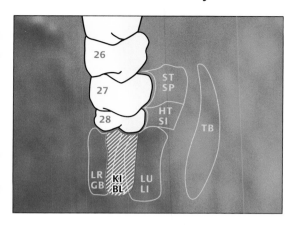

The vestibular points correlated to the kidney–bladder network are situated opposite the crowns of the incisor teeth of upper and lower jaw, right and left.

"Kidney–bladder zones" in the retromolar space are projected

a) in the upper jaw: distally of the tuber maxillae,

a) in the lower jaw: lingually in the retromolar space.

Therapy Options

► Urogenital dysfunctions and disorders

► Lumbar spine and iliosacral joint conditions

► "Chill disorders"

Effects of oral acupuncture as well as results of electroacupuncture tests have confirmed that the so-called "*yang* kidney"—including the adrenals—is represented within the retromolar "kidney zone."

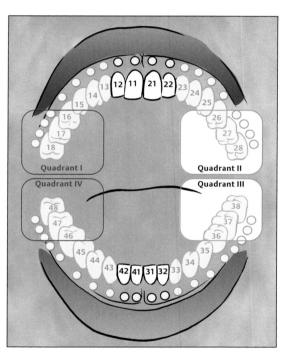

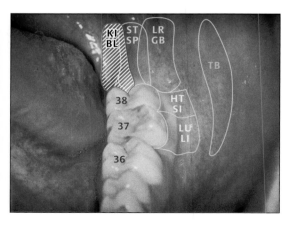

Functional Network: Liver–Gallbladder

The vestibular points correlated to the liver–gall-bladder network are situated opposite the crowns of the canine teeth of upper and lower jaw, right and left.

"Liver–gallbladder zones" in the retromolar space are projected

a) in the upper jaw: palatally in the retromolar space,
a) in the lower jaw: buccally in the retromolar space.

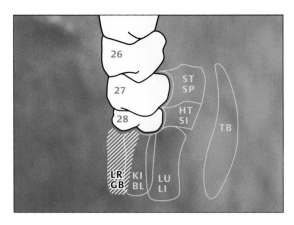

Therapy Options

► Digestive and metabolic conditions

► Joint disorders, particularly of hip and knee

► Restricted movement owing to muscle spasms and shortenings

► Migraine

► Vertigo, dizziness

► Eye disorders

► Overemotional behavior

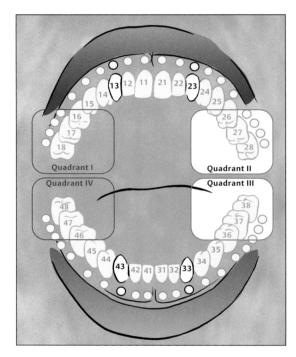

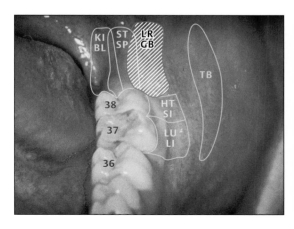

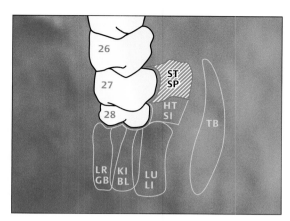

Functional Network: Spleen/Pancreas–Stomach

The vestibular points correlated to the spleen–stomach network are situated

a) in the upper jaw: adjacent to molar teeth (O-16/O-17; O-26/O-27),

b) in the lower jaw: adjacent to premolar teeth (O-34/O-35; O-44/O-45).

"Spleen/pancreas–stomach zones" are to be found in the middle section of the retromolar spaces, especially in the lower jaw.

Therapy Options

► Gastrointestinal complaints, maldigestion

► Lymphatic and allergic disorders

► Dysfunction of the connective tissue

► Pasty swellings

► Worrying behavior

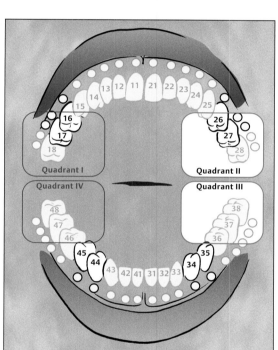

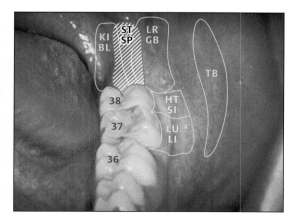

236

Functional Network:
Lung–Large Intestine

The vestibular points correlated to the lung–large intestine network are situated

a) in the upper jaw: adjacent to premolar teeth (O-14/O-15; O-24/O-25),

b) in the lower jaw: adjacent to molar teeth (O-36/O-37; O-46/O-47).

NOTE *This is vice versa to the localization of spleen points.*

"Lung–large intestine zones" are to be found buccally in the retromolar space, especially of the upper jaw.

Therapy Options

► Dysfunctions and infections of the respiratory system, bronchitis, bronchial asthma, sinusitis, and rhinitis

► Intestinal complaints, dysbiosis of the microflora

► Shoulder and elbow complaints (preferably use upper jaw points)

► Hypersensitivity (environmental conditions)

► Hopelessness

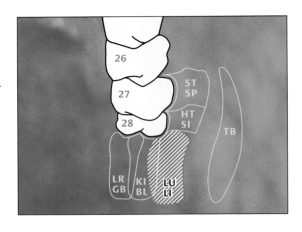

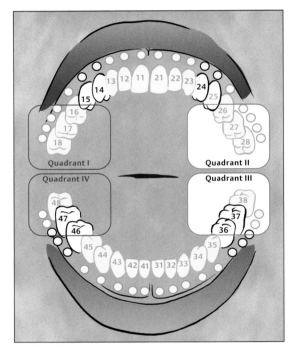

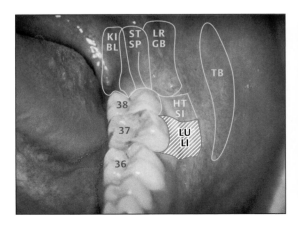

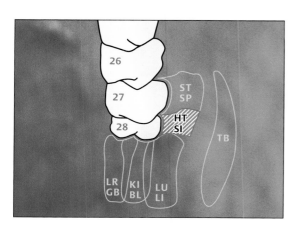

Functional Network: Heart–Small Intestine

The vestibular points correlated to the heart–small intestine network are situated adjacent to the wisdom teeth, i.e., next to the mucobuccal fold (O-18; O-28; O-38; O-48).

The wisdom teeth area is the link between vestibular and retromolar point systems.

Therapy Options

► Functional heart complaints

► Digestive disorders

► Psychosomatic and vegetative conditions

► Pain conditions and swellings at the contralateral wisdom tooth area (dentitio difficilis, postoperative pain etc)

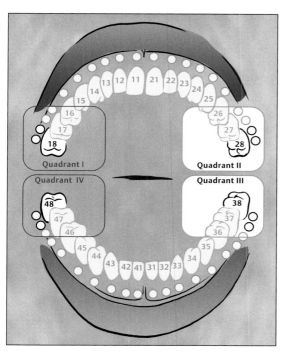

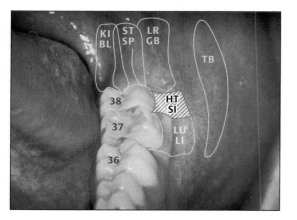

Oral Acupuncture

Triple Burner–Pericardium Channels

There is no assignment to vestibulum points. The Triple Burner is represented at the front edge of the ascending mandibula. This area has to be palpated carefully by pressing the finger tip against the frontal edge of the ascending mandible, gliding upward from the linea obliqua: the Triple Burner points are found halfway between the upper and lower jaw. The pericardium channel seems to be projected at identical points.

Therapy Options

- ► Migraine
- ► Spasms
- ► Headache
- ► Neurohormonal dysregulations

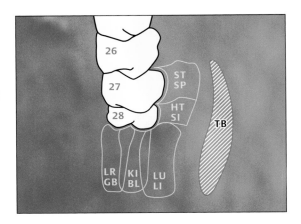

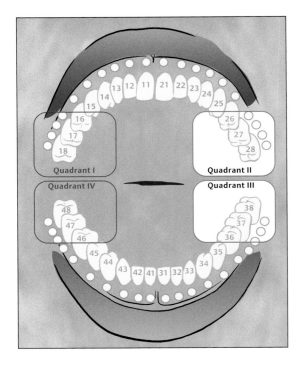

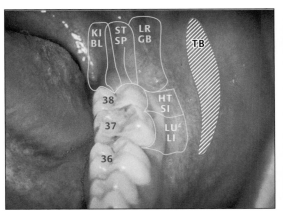

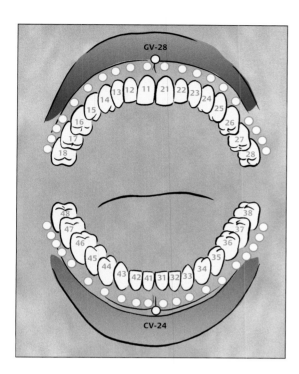

Frenular Points

These points have to be detected at either side of the frenula.

Therapy Options

► Local affections of oral mucous membrane, for example, gingivitis, stomatitis

► Upper jaw frenular points: Anal disorders such as hemorrhoids, anal fissures; spinal complaints

► Lower jaw frenular points: Urogenital disorders, *yin* deficiency complaints

Extraoral Points

Extraoral points of special importance are to be found close to the outer edge of the lips. Their location is derived from the analogous enoral points suggesting a perforating needle. Point detection is preferably performed by the "very-point" technique (see p. 242) i.e. dabbing the acupuncture needle tangentially across the skin, parallel to the lip in a distance of one centimeter.

Therapy Options

► The extraoral point analogous to the enoral canine point proved very effective in treatment of hip and knee complaints.

Oral Acupuncture

Musculoskeletal System

The respective joints and parts of the musculoskeletal systems can be treated by points correlated to their respective segments and channels.

For *temporomandibular joint:* Use points that may relax the pterygoid muscles: the lateral pterygoid muscle may respond to point treatment buccally/distally in the upper jaw retromolar space; the medial pterygoid muscle may respond to treatment lingually in the lower jaw retromolar space.

Cervical spine: Atlas and axis including their inserting muscles and tendons can be treated effectively by retromolar points of the lower jaw. The lower sections of the cervical spine, the cervicothoracic junctions, as well as the *thoracic spine* can best be treated by palatal retromolar points of the upper jaw.

The *lumbar spine* is represented buccally in the lower wisdom teeth in an area extending towards the retromolar area of the lower jaw.

The *iliosacral joint* is represented lingually in the retromolar area of the lower jaw, next to the "Kidney–bladder zone."

For *shoulder–elbow* complaints, use points situated buccally and distally in the retromolar area of the upper jaw.

Hip and knee complaints are preferably treated by vestibular points, that is, by canine points of the lower jaw (O-39/O-49).

In the list above, preference has been attributed rather to retromolar points because these are generally superior in treatment. Vestibular points are prior in diagnosis. However, they may be treated additionally if therapy in the retromolar space proves unsatisfactory.

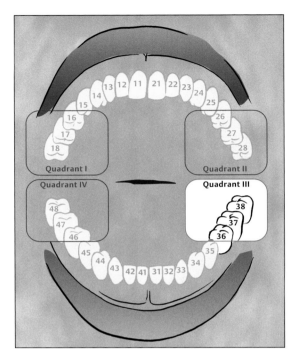

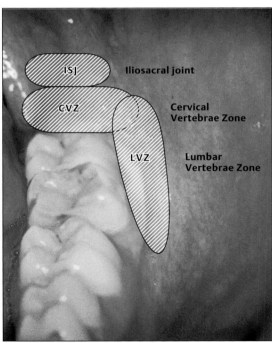

Correlations of the spinal column and of the iliosacral joint

Pain Management

Oral Acupuncture has also proved effective in the case of trigeminal neuralgia and other kinds of orofacial pain. For frontal sinusitis cephalgia, use points of kidney–bladder correlation. For orofacial pain affecting the nasal and labial areas, use points of spleen–stomach resp. lung–large intestine correlation.

In cases of excruciating pain—such as trigeminal neuralgia—treatment must only be applied contralaterally to the afflicted area. In this case, exactly symmetrical points must be detected both in the face and enorally. Any local pain condition of the stomatognathic system can be treated via analogous points sharing the same network correlation. This applies to points of the contralateral jaws, of the counter-jaw, as well as to retromolar points of the afflicted quadrant.

In case of long-standing conditions, it is advisable to search for scars in the affected quadrant. If such relicts of earlier injuries prove sensitive to instrumental detection, the scars should be injected with a local anesthetic.

Practical Instructions

In general, the *rule of homolaterality* applies to Oral Acupuncture. For instance, complaints on the left side are treated via the Oral Acupuncture points on the left. In chronic illnesses, however, bilateral injections have proved beneficial. In acute pain conditions, symmetrical therapy is applicable (see above).

Therapy prerogatives are:

1. Optimum illumination

2. Firm support of the patient's head

3. Inspection of the entire mucous membrane in order to register local inflammation, aphtha, ulcers, etc.

4. Examination by palpation and/or instrumental detection

5. Administration of injection using a low-percentage local anesthetic (0.5% without addition of a vasoconstrictor). Allergy to the local anesthetic in question must be ruled out.

Treatment should be limited to only three to six points per session. This helps to avoid an initial worsening of symptoms. This kind of over-reaction may occur especially following the first session. However, it indicates that the patient's self-regulatory systems have been stimulated successfully.

Treatment may be administered using vestibular points or retromolar points. Retromolar points, however, have proved to be superior in therapy; treatment of retromolar points, if successful, will probably deactivate vestibular points immediately so that these are "deleted." This "extinguishing" phenomenon indicates a certain hierarchy because it only works one way. Hierarchies are a common feature in system theory.

In cases of nonresponders to oral acupuncture, other microsystems and/or traditional acupuncture must be included.

Oral Acupuncture

Point Detection

Oral points, if indicated for therapy, show a higher degree of sensitivity. Therefore, palpation is an important feature in Oral Acupuncture. The points chosen for treatment have to be precisely localized. Digital palpation, of course, can only give rough hints. Bioelectric detectors do not work in the oral cavity because of the moisture of the mucous membranes. For exact spotting, therefore, detection by means of an instrument with a fine tip is necessary, e.g. using a fine ball probe (as used by dentists for fillings).

Most precise localization can be achieved by using the injection needle itself as a detection instrument ("very point" technique). For this purpose, the needle has to be handled very gently, dabbing it gradually and tangentially in a non-traumatizing manner across the suspect area. At the selfsame moment when the "very point" is hit, the patient will invariably respond with an unmistakable facial expression and/or a verbal affirmation. At this instant, the needle must be slightly erected and inserted.

The "very point" technique was developed to meet the special conditions of Oral Acupuncture. However, it is also applicable at skin points.

Therapy by Injection

Oral Acupuncture is best administered by means of injections, as the use of needles in the oral cavity is dangerous. Only the finest disposable cannulas and preferably insulin or tuberculin syringes are to be used, or very fine dental cannulas.

Local anesthetics of low percentage (0.2–0.5%) have proved most effective in Oral Acupuncture. Instead, physiological sodium-chloride solution or homeopathic remedies may be used as well. The quantity of local anesthetic used should be kept as low as possible. It is not the amount of injection fluid that matters but hitting the exact point. As a rule, it will be sufficient to inject two to four drops per point. After injection, the bubble should be dispersed by digital massage.

Use of Laser

Low-level laser acupuncture has proved suitable in Oral Acupuncture because it is painless, an important feature in the treatment of hypersensitive patients. Overstimulation must be avoided at any rate. No more than four to six points should be treated per session. The duration of irradiation depends on the output of the device.

Electrostimulation is contraindicated in the oral cavity.

Side Effects

If treatment is performed lege artis, adverse side-effects are most unlikely. Initial deterioration may occur. It is indicative of onsetting regulation.

Caution is required when treating patients who are receiving anticoagulative therapy.

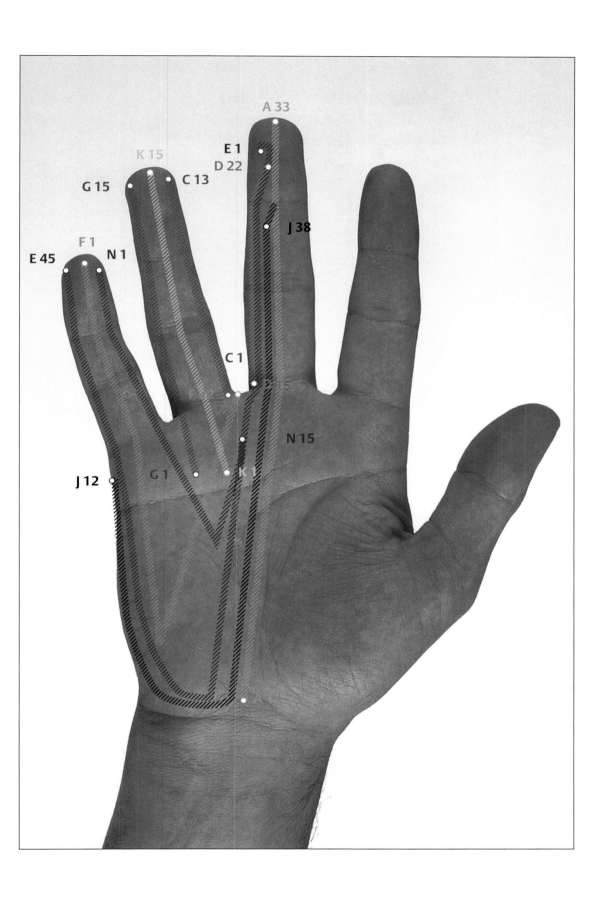

Hand Acupuncture Points on the Palm of the Hand

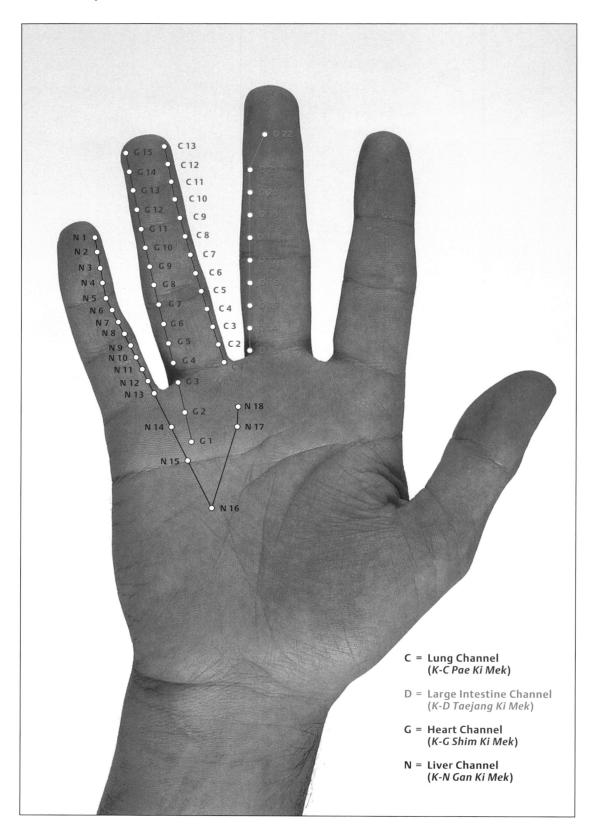

C = **Lung Channel**
(*K-C Pae Ki Mek*)

D = Large Intestine Channel
(*K-D Taejang Ki Mek*)

G = **Heart Channel**
(*K-G Shim Ki Mek*)

N = **Liver Channel**
(*K-N Gan Ki Mek*)

The K-A Im Ki Mek corresponds to the Conception Vessel of body acupuncture and runs straight along the centerline on the palm of the hand—corresponding to the third digit. It starts at A 1 (5 mm distal to the center of the distal flexion crease of the wrist) and ends at A 33 (2 mm proximal to the nail) on the middle finger. In contrast to body acupuncture, the Governing Vessel is represented from the upper lip to the parting (GV-26–GV-20) by the Governing Vessel (A 26–A 33) in hand acupuncture. The points on the palm of the hand, likewise on the middle finger, are proportionally allocated, i.e. they are found by dividing in half each time (cf. illustration on left: e.g. point A 8—navel—is located precisely halfway between points A 1 and A 16).

The K-A Im Ki Mek plays an important role in both the diagnosis and treatment of diseases. Most alarm points, i.e. those points which indicate the condition of the corresponding organ, are located on the Conception Vessel. It is the "Sea of all *Yin* Channels" and like the Governing Vessel and the *chong mai* ("Thoroughfare Vessel"), obtains its energy from the kidneys and, consequently, has a link to the essences. Its chief significance is for the reproductive system, as it controls fertility, menstruation, pregnancy, and menopause. Individual points lead in particular to a strengthening of the *yin* or the *yin* organs and are therefore used in particular for vacuity–heat symptoms in the Lower Burner, but also in the Middle and Upper Burner. The Conception Vessel (Im Ki Mek) has its opposite number in the Governing Vessel (Dok Ki Mek), which explains the positive effect obtained by needling the corresponding area of the lower abdomen (A 1–A 8) in cases of deep, median lumbago—according to the front-to-back rule.

Refresher: Important points of K-A Im Ki Mek

⊙ **A 1:** Sexual organs, psychosexual disorders

⊙ **A 3:** Bladder diseases, main energy point for men

⊙ **A 4:** Small intestine alarm point, uterus, and main energy point for women

⊙ **A 5:** Triple Burner alarm point, all gynecological disorders

⊙ **A 8:** Navel, controls congenital and acquired life functions

⊙ **A 12:** Stomach alarm point, used in basic treatment with Middle Burner

⊙ **A 16:** Heart alarm point

⊙ **A 18:** Pericardium alarm point, main point for all thorax complaints, important point of the upper burner

⊙ **A 20:** Larynx, pharynx, and gullet pain

⊙ **A 28:** Nasal diseases

⊙ **A 33:** Mental illnesses, headaches, and unconsciousness. Important point for shock, epilepsy, diarrhea (needling of this point draws the *qi* upwards—thus counteracts the sinking of weak spleen *qi*)

Korean Hand Acupuncture

Governing Vessel: K-B Dok Ki Mek

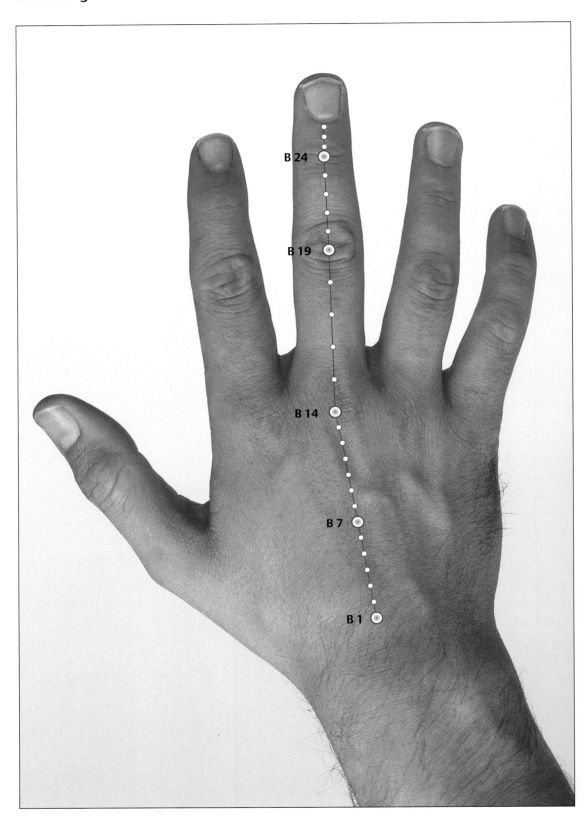

The K-B Dok Ki Mek corresponds to the Governing Vessel of body acupuncture and runs straight along the centerline on the back of the hand (corresponding to the third digit) opposite the K-A Im Ki Mek. It starts at B 1 (5 mm distal to the center of the wrist) and ends at B 27 (2 mm proximal to the nail bed) on the middle finger.

The K-B Dok Ki Mek is the "Sea of *Yang*" and strengthens the *yang* of the whole body. It strengthens the spinal column and the whole skeletal musculature via the kidney *yang* and thus influences complaints in the region of the spinal column and head. In addition, it regulates the circulation of blood to the brain and the performance of the brain, for which reason it is treated in cases of reduced mental capacity and apoplexy. Several points in particular strengthen the *yang*, namely B 7 (corresponding to GV-4) and B 19 (corresponding to GV-14).

Refresher: Important points of K-B Dok Ki Mek

○ **B 1:** Anal diseases, coccyx complaints, chronic lumbago, cramps of the extremities, and unconsciousness

○ **B 7:** Corresponds to GV-4; for general debility, kidney weakness, chronic lumbago, kindles life fire, impotence, navel pain (front–back coupling)

○ **B 14:** Heart disease

○ **B 19:** Relaxes the whole nape of the neck–shoulder region, strengthens *yang*, indication for diseases of the head, face, throat, chest area, and the digestive organs

○ **B 24:** Diseases of the head, face, back, and nerves in mental illnesses; in apoplexy and unconsciousness

Lung Channel: K-C Pae Ki Mek

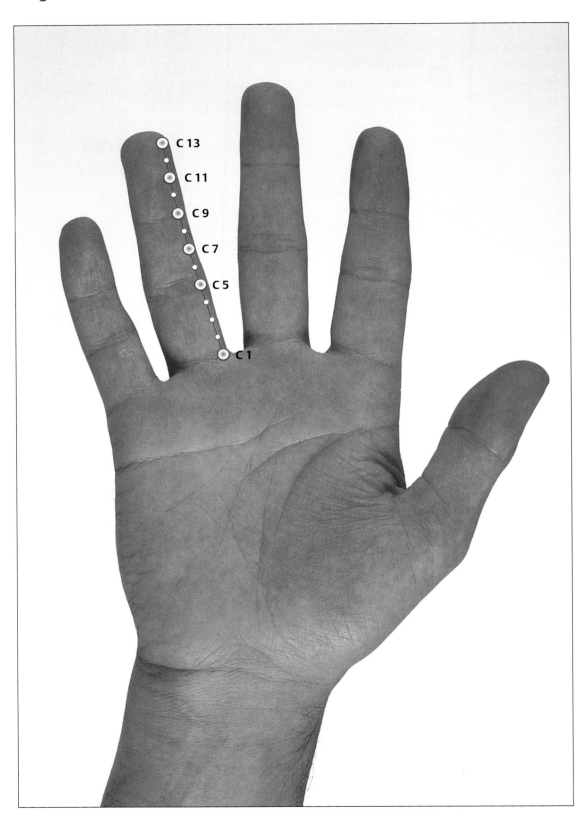

The lung obtains its energy from food via spleen *qi* and from *ate wei qi*. On the hand, K-C Pae Ki Mek arises at the base joint of the ring finger on the radial side and stretches along the radial side of the finger to the tip of the nail.

Refresher: Important points of K-C Pae Ki Mek

⊙ **C 1:** In all lung diseases, skin diseases, helps distinguish between symptoms of deficiency and excess

⊙ **C 5:** Entry point of lung energy to the channel, reduces fullness in the event of symptoms of excess of the lung

⊙ **C 7:** Cardinal point of the Lung Channel, switches on K-A Im Ki Mek; point at which lung energy flows particularly strongly, together with J 2 strengthens *yin*; together with K-I Bang-Kwang Ki Mek strengthens bladder function

⊙ **C 9:** Source point, used for tonification of the Lung Channel, controls the blood vessels and the pulse, purifies lung and liver–heat symptoms

⊙ **C 11:** For bronchitis and asthma, dispels symptoms of wind

⊙ **C 13:** For acute lung diseases, for symptoms of lung excess

Large Intestine Channel: K-D Taejang Ki Mek

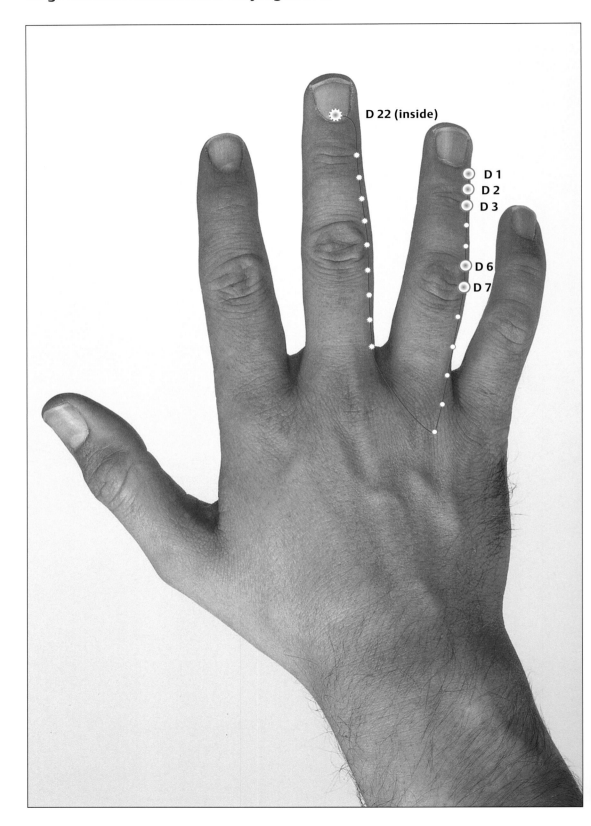

D 22 (inside)

D 1
D 2
D 3

D 6
D 7

The Large Intestine Channel is the complementary *yang* channel to the Lung Channel. It influences all intestinal diseases from the end of the small intestine to the anus. Frequently, however, diseases of the stomach and duodenum are also better treated via the Large Intestine Channel. In the case of a *yang* constitution, excess of the large intestine is chiefly responsible for complaints. Lumbago in the region of L4/5 with typical pressure pain at the alarm point of the large intestine E 22 (= ST-25) is therefore treated by sedating the large intestine.

The K-D Taejang Ki Mek begins on the outside corner of the nail of the ring finger and stretches along the ulnar edge of the finger to the base joint. At D 12 it changes course, twines around the metacarpal capitulum, and runs along the ulnar side of the middle finger to the ungual phalanx, where it ends at D 22 to the side of the nose equivalent.

> ### Refresher: Important points of K-D Taejang Ki Mek
>
> ⊙ **D 1:** For digestive problems, stomach aches, headaches, toothache
>
> ⊙ **D 2:** Most important point for large intestine excess, intestinal problems, toothache
>
> ⊙ **D 3:** For all chronic intestinal complaints, facial pain, dispels internal wind, for wind–heat symptoms, acute conjunctivitis, in the initial stages of a chill
>
> ⊙ **D 6:** Controls function of the large intestine; additional, important point for large intestine hyperactivity, for lung *qi* weakness with immune deficiency, for shoulder pain
>
> ⊙ **D 7:** Gateway of channel energy to the intestine, used for acute diseases such as acute tonsillitis, sore throat, acute pain along the channel
>
> ⊙ **D 22:** Rhinitis, toothache, as a local point for facial pain

Korean Hand Acupuncture

Stomach Channel: K-E Wie Ki Mek

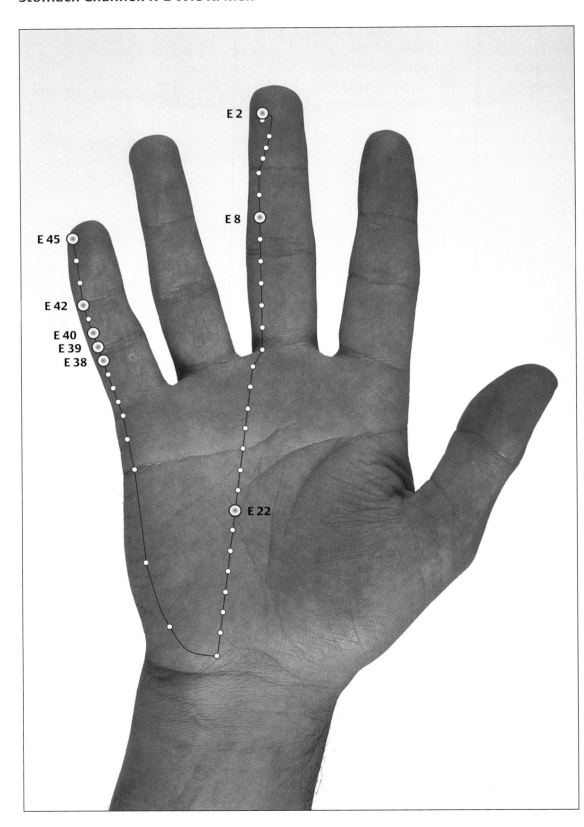

As a *yang* channel, the Stomach Channel together with its *yin*-coupled channel, the Spleen Channel, controls digestion. In TCM, the digestion plays a central role in the provision of *qi* and blood and is therefore also regarded as a storehouse of food *qi* in the *Nei King*. A weak digestion therefore gives rise to a weak immune system and as an additional consequence, weakness of all body functions. The Stomach Channel, in accordance with its course, regulates the function of the eyes, the facial musculature, the digestion, and potency. Stomach *qi* tends to decline. In the event of malfunction, it increases and symptoms such as nausea, sickness, hiccups, heartburn, defective vision, nervous eye tic, etc. are the result.

K-E Wie Ki Mek begins at the tip of the middle finger (E 1), then stretches diagonally outward to the ulnar end of the flexion crease of the distal interphalangeal joint (E 6), runs parallel to K-A Im Ki Mek to the base joint flexion crease (E 14), continues over the palm of the hand approx. 5 mm next to K-A Im Ki Mek to E 29 (next to A 1), bends at a right angle, and runs along the edge of the hand and then on the outside of the little finger to the outer nail tip, where it ends at point E 45 (ST-45).

Refresher: Important points of K-E Wie Ki Mek

⊙ **E 2:** Eye problems, upper jaw pain

⊙ **E 8:** In-Yong = Carotid Point (important for pulse diagnosis), throat–pharynx problems, goiter

⊙ **E 2:** Alarm point of the large intestine

⊙ **E 38:** Knee pain at the front, gateway of K-E Wie Ki Mek

⊙ **E 39:** Earth point of the Stomach Channel, strengthens *qi* and blood, controls stomach–spleen function, strengthens defense *qi*, helps in cases of disturbed appetite, dispels wind, dampness, and cold, flushes out edema

⊙ **E 40:** Shoulder pain, controls stomach function

⊙ **E 42:** Source point, strengthens spleen and stomach, calms the mind, ankle joint complaints

⊙ **E 45:** The point at which the channel energy arises, helps with all acute stomach problems, main point for upset stomach (microphlebotomy), stomach ulcer, stomach bleeding

Spleen Channel: K-F Pi Ki Mek

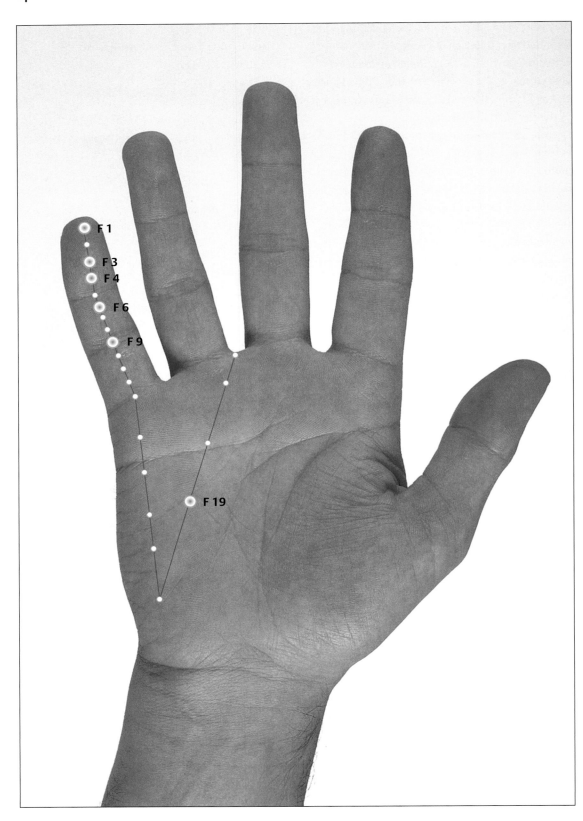

The spleen lies in the center of the body and, together with the stomach, represents the central digestive organ. In the *Nei King*, the spleen is described as the basis, the determining organ for all the internal organs. Man requires a fixed, grounded base in order to ward off disease. If the spleen is vacuous, man becomes prone to disease—there is a loss of appetite, a tendency to diarrhea, general weakness, and cachexia. Mental strain, for example as a result of excessive study, brooding, and worry, weakens the spleen–pancreas. If the spleen–pancreas is in excess, the patient tends to obesity, constipation, and diabetes.

The Spleen Channel starts in the center of the tip of the little finger, extends precisely in the middle on the volar side to the center of the base joint flexion crease, continues across the hypothenar and across the base of MC* V (F 18), turns almost in the opposite direction, and runs slightly diagonally across the palm of the hand to F 22, on the side at the end of the flexion crease of the base joint of the middle finger.

* MC=metarcarpal (bone)

Refresher: Important points of K-F Pi Ki Mek

⊙ **F 1:** For digestive disturbances, strengthens the spleen, regulates the blood, stops bleeding, calms the mind

⊙ **F 3:** Source point of the channel, strengthens spleen *qi* in all forms of weakness, especially effective in cases of weakness of the spleen as a result of mental strain, dries spleen dampness

⊙ **F 4:** Cardinal point, for heart disease, lower abdominal pain, dysmenorrhea, endometritis, digestive weakness—food lies in the stomach

⊙ **F 6:** "Sea of Lower Yin Channels," important point for all diseases of sexual organs, menopausal complaints

⊙ **F 9:** Knee pain, urogenital diseases, excess fluid in the body

⊙ **F 19:** Spleen alarm point, stomach pain, back pain, epilepsy

Korean Hand Acupuncture

Heart Channel: K-G Shim Ki Mek

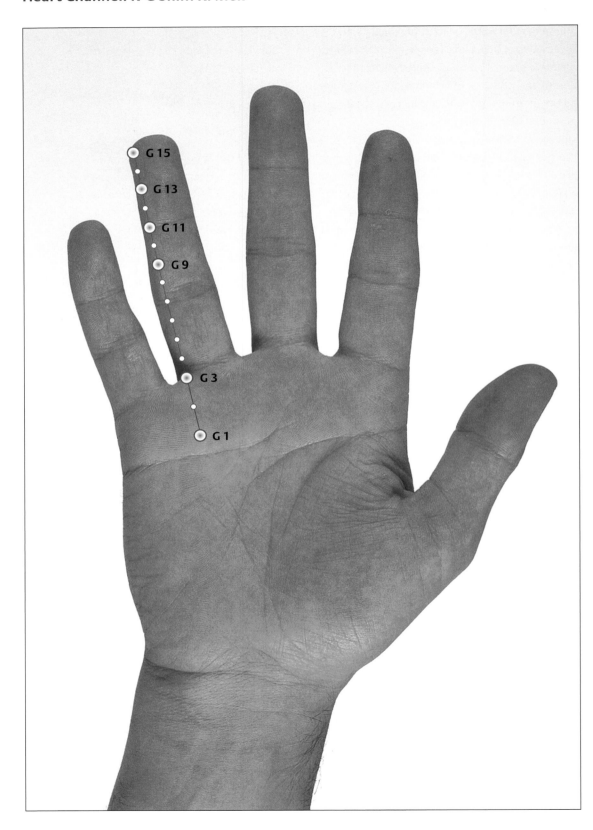

In TCM the most important tasks of the heart are to govern the blood and the spirit—the performance of the brain. Blood and *yin* are the sources of the spirit. Thus, a healthy heart results in a clear, pure spirit which is reflected in a bright, shining face. If the heart is weak, the face is pale, flaccid, and ugly—the spirit is likewise weak and tired and the patient feels unhappy and depressed. As the heart opens at the tongue, speech problems such as motor aphasia, stuttering, or rapid, delirious speech are always indications of heart disease.

K-G Shim Ki Mek arises at G 1 in the palm of the hand on the ulnar side of the capitulum of MC IV and extends along the edge of the ring finger on the side of the little finger to the tip of the nail on the side at Point G 15.

> **Refresher: Important points of K-G Shim Ki Mek**
>
> ⊙ **G 1:** Mental anxiety, cramps, diarrhea, sickness in small children
>
> ⊙ **G 3:** As above, sedates heart–fire, calms the mind
>
> ⊙ **G 7:** Connecting point at which the channel energy flows into the heart, important in small children together with G 1 and G 3 for cramps (microphlebotomy), vacuity heat of the heart, hypertension, heart disease, pain in the thorax
>
> ⊙ **G 9:** At this point the heart energy flows into K-G Shim Ki Mek, for heart *qi* weakness, mental illness, pain in the thorax, disturbed rhythms
>
> ⊙ **G 11:** Source point of K-G Shim Ki Mek, "Gateway of the Mind," for all heart disease, for all neurasthenic complaints, mental illness, insomnia, calms the mind, for paralyses, and for cramps in small children
>
> ⊙ **G 13:** Fire Point, for all heat disorders, vacuity fire, mucus fire
>
> ⊙ **G 15:** End point of K-G Shim Ki Mek, emergency point for cramps, collapse, unconsciousness

Korean Hand Acupuncture

Small Intestine Channel: K-H Sojang Ki Mek

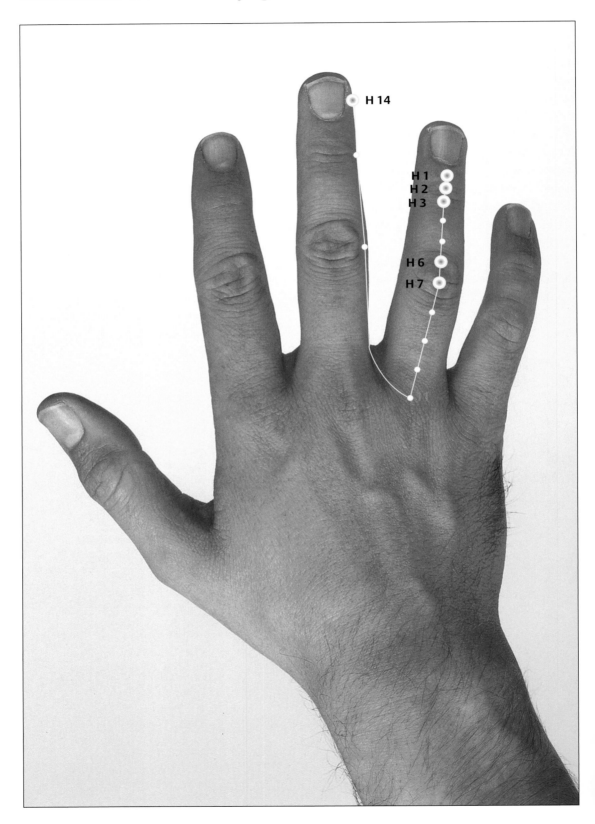

The small intestine is the *yang* organ associated with the heart. It is nourished by the stomach–spleen, separates impure fluids, sends these to the bladder, and conveys unusable food components to the large intestine.

K-H Sojang Ki Mek arises in the middle of the nail bed of the ring finger, runs to the base joint in the centerline at H 11, and turns to the middle finger, where it extends precisely along the side to the center of the nail of the middle finger at H 14.

Refresher: Important points of K-H Sojang Ki Mek

⊙ **H 1:** In the acute stage of rheumatism, angina tonsillaris, laryngitis, headaches in the occiput, particularly if these are the result of a wind–heat attack from outside. It also opens up the channel to eliminate internal wind, e.g. in apoplexy as a result of internal wind

⊙ **H 2:** Cardinal point, switches on K-B Dok Ki Mek, nape of the neck, shoulder, pain in the vertebral column, beneficial effect on all muscles and tendons along the Governor Vessel, and the Bladder and Small Intestine Channel, with regard to wind–heat the same applies as for H 1

⊙ **H 3:** Regulates the Small Intestine Channel, for heart *qi* weakness

⊙ **H 6:** For diseases of the large intestine and stomach

⊙ **H 7:** Earth point, reduces fullness of small intestine, swelling of the lymph nodes in the nape of the neck, parotitis, pain in the nape of the neck, shoulder blades, elbows, and back

⊙ **H 14:** Tinnitus, otitis, trigeminal neuralgia

Korean Hand Acupuncture

Bladder Channel: K-I Bang-Kwang Ki Mek

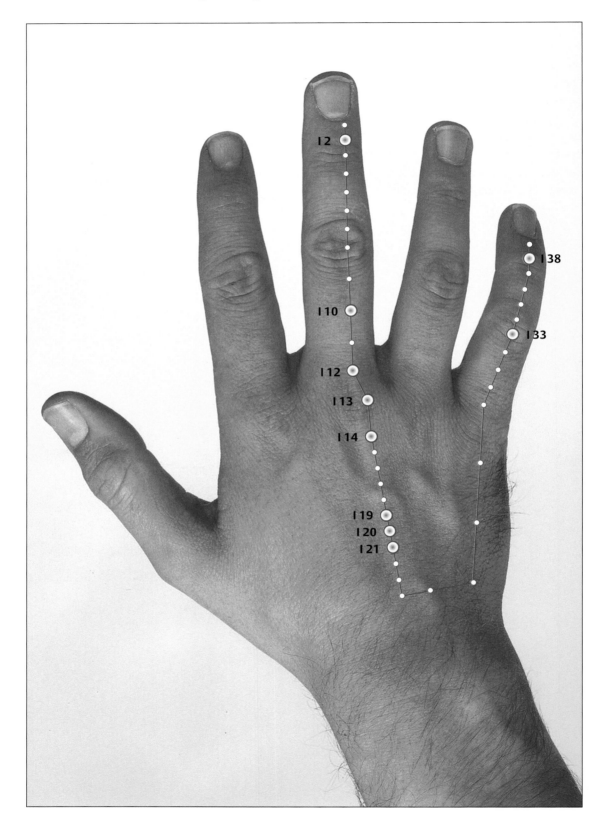

The bladder stores the impure fluids that are excreted by the kidney. As the longest channel, it extends from the eyes over the head and nape of the neck, on either side of the spinal column over the back to the buttocks, and continues across the back of the legs to the little toe. Its route explains its influence on the eyes, the head, the back, and lumbar region, as well as the lower extremities. The major significance of the Bladder Channel is also evident from the fact that all the consent points of the organs are located on it.

K-I Bang-Kwang Ki Mek begins in the nail bed of the middle finger with I 1, runs along the side of K-B Dok Ki Mek on the back of the hand in the direction of the wrist, turns at I 24 in an ulnar direction, extends to the little finger at the fifth digit, and ends two millimeters before the nail bed at I 39.

> **Refresher: Important points of K-I Bang-Kwang Ki Mek**
>
> ⊙ **I 2:** Pain in the occiput–nape of the neck, vertigo, vertebral artery equivalent point
>
> ⊙ **I 10:** Lung consent point
>
> ⊙ **I 12:** Heart consent point
>
> ⊙ **I 13:** Relaxes the diaphragm
>
> ⊙ **I 14:** Liver consent point
>
> ⊙ **I 19:** Kidney consent point
>
> ⊙ **I 20:** Large intestine consent point
>
> ⊙ **I 21:** Small intestine consent point
>
> ⊙ **I 33:** Back of the knee, controls Bladder Channel energy, thins the blood, relaxes the tendons
>
> ⊙ **I 38:** Important point for fullness of the bladder, one of the famous eight points (Pal Sung Hyul), cardinal or intervention points of the extraordinary channels

Kidney Channel: K-J Shin Ki Mek

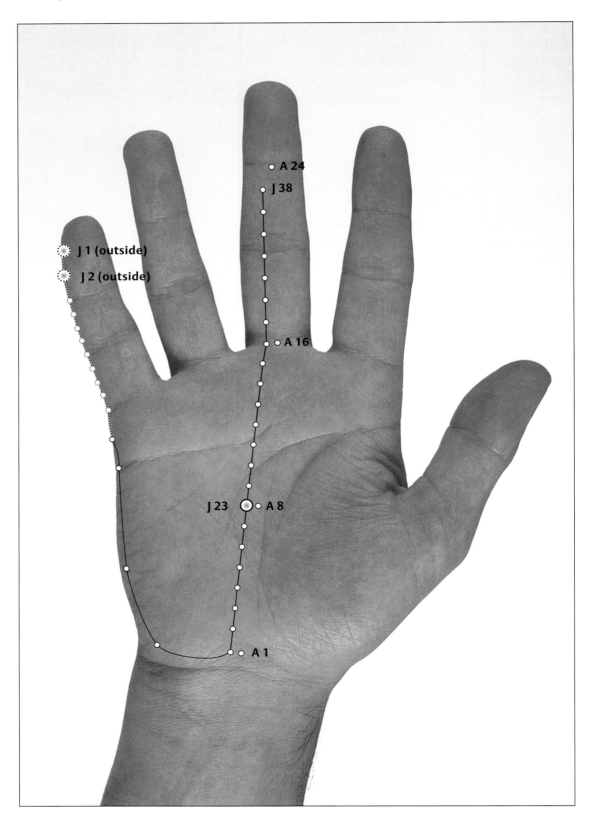

The kidney has a special place in TCM. It is the root of vital energy and stores the essences, the *jing*. The *yin* kidney symbolizes the water kidney, the *yang* kidney the fire kidney (adrenal gland). In contrast to TCM acupuncture, in Korean hand acupuncture the water kidney is also consciously sedated (*sin* constitution).

K-J Shin Ki Mek arises at the outer corner of the nail of the little finger at J 1, runs along the outside edge of the little finger to J 11, turns on the volar side, and extends parallel to K-A Im Ki Mek to the pharyngeal space on the middle joint of the middle finger (J 38).

> **Refresher: Important points of K-J Shin Ki Mek**
>
> ⊙ **J 1:** Origin of channel energy, emergency point as opener to earth, pharyngitis, tonsillitis
>
> ⊙ **J 2:** Strengthens kidney *yin* and *yang*, cardinal point, cough
>
> ⊙ **J 23:** Alarm point of the kidneys, for kidney fullness, swelling in the navel region

Pericardium Channel: K-K Shim-Po Ki Mek

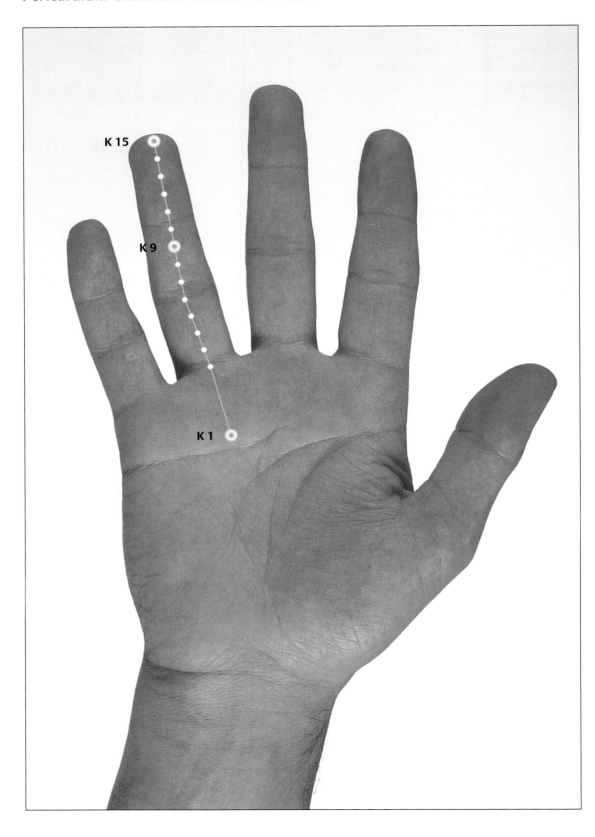

The Pericardium Channel governs blood flow in conjunction with the heart and is sensitive to external, pathogenic influences instead of the Heart Channel. Together with the Triple Burner, it influences all complaints in the region of the thorax and upper abdomen.

K-K Shim-Po Ki Mek begins in the palm of the hand in the region of the capitulum of MC IV and extends in the center of the ring finger to the fingertip K 15.

> **Refresher: Important points of K-K Shim-Po Ki Mek**
>
> ⊙ **K 1:** For chronic digestive complaints
>
> ⊙ **K 9:** Cardinal point for all *yin* organs, relieves the thorax, for nausea and sickness, important point together with A 18 for toothache
>
> ⊙ **K 15:** End point and emergency point for unconsciousness

Triple Burner Channel: K-L Sam-Cho Ki Mek

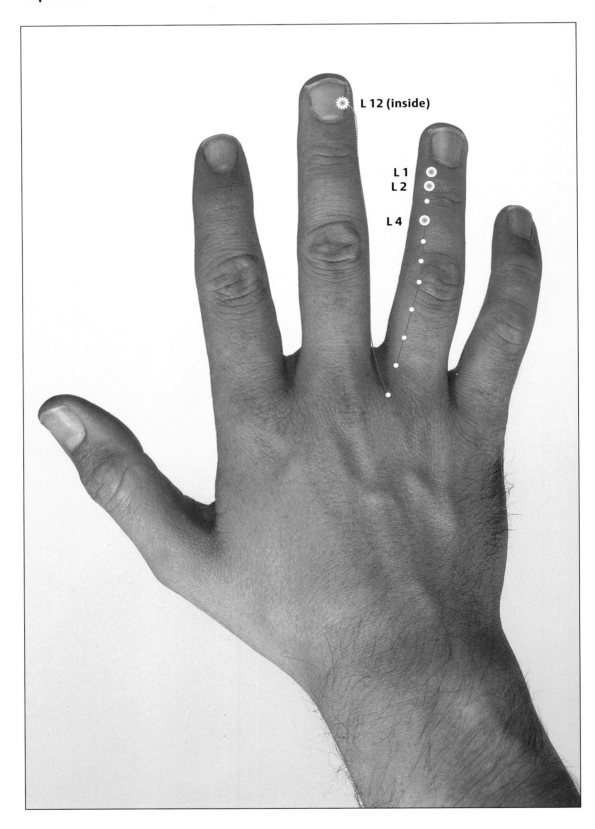

No substantial organ corresponds to the Triple Burner, but it regulates the functions of the organs of the three abdominal cavities. It serves to open up the energy flows in the channels.

K-L Sam-Cho Ki Mek begins at the corner of the nail of the ring finger on the side nearest the middle finger, extends sideways to the metacarpophalangeal joint L 11, turns to the side of the middle finger, and ends with L 12 at the level of the ear on the ungual phalanx.

> **Refresher: Important points of K-L Sam-Cho Ki Mek**
>
> ⊙ **L 1:** Origin point of the channel energy, for Triple Burner fullness, unconsciousness
>
> ⊙ **L 2:** Headaches, otitis, shoulder blade–nape of the neck pain
>
> ⊙ **L 4:** Cardinal point for *yang* organs, rheumatism, migraine, facial paresis
>
> ⊙ **L 12:** Cephalgia, facial pain

Gallbladder Channel: K-M Dam Ki Mek

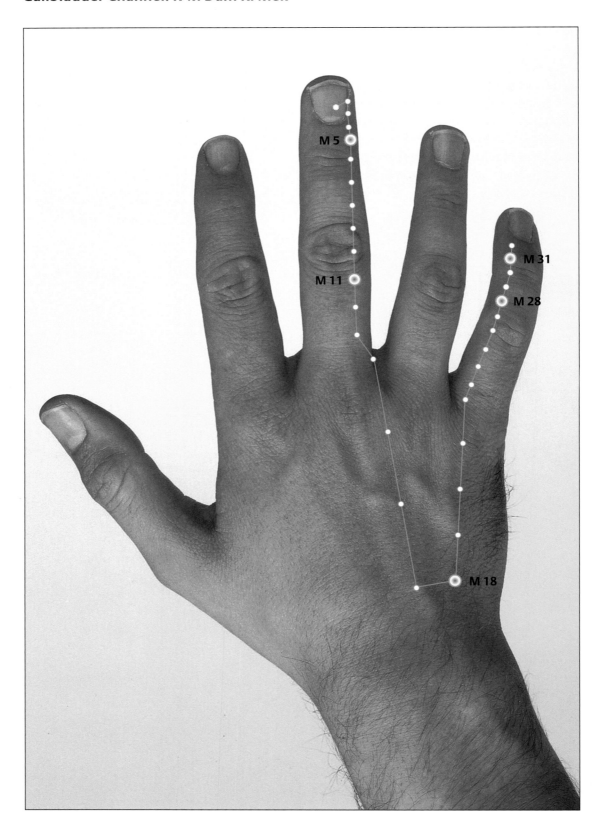

The Gallbladder Channel is related to the lateral side of the body. It is the opposite number of the Liver Channel and governs the joints and tendons. Wind, as an external, pathogenic, bioclimatic factor, affects the Gallbladder Channel in particular.

K-M Dam Ki Mek begins at the tip of the nail of the middle finger on the side with M 1, runs along the edge of the middle finger and across the back of the hand to the wrist (M 17), turns, and extends along the fifth digit to the corner of the nail of the little finger (M 32).

Refresher: Important points of K-M Dam Ki Mek

⊙ **M 5:** Pain on the side of the neck, neuralgia, hypertension, apoplexy

⊙ **M 11:** Shoulder blade and neck pain

⊙ **M 18:** Together with M 20, M 21, M 22 for hip and hip joint pain

⊙ **M 28:** General analgesic point

⊙ **M 31:** Cardinal point of dai mai (belt vessel), knee and hip pain

Korean Hand Acupuncture

Liver Channel: K-N Gan Ki Mek

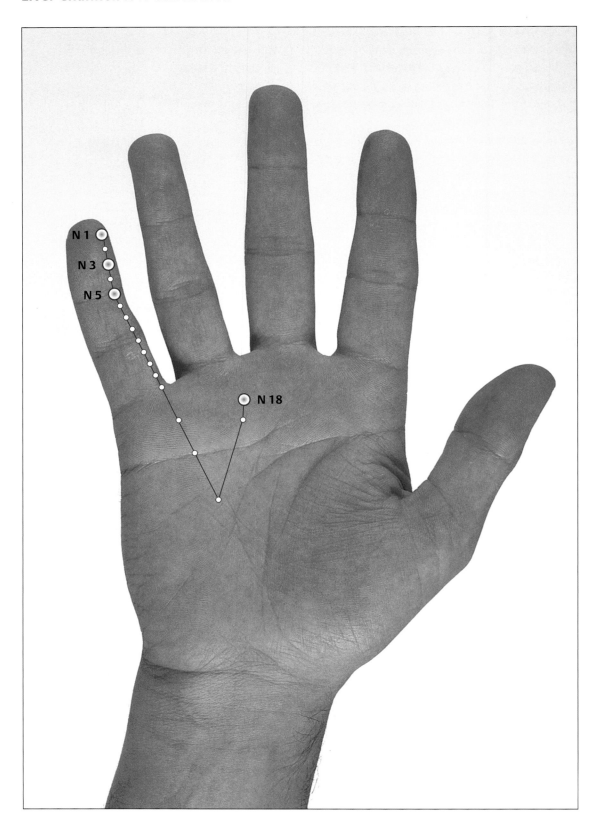

The main task of the liver is to ensure the smooth flow of *qi* in all organs. It safeguards the flow of *qi* particularly in the sexual organs and, therefore, regulates menstruation and fertility. As the seat of the soul, it has an important relationship with the emotions and, therefore, with mental illness. As the liver pumps its blood to the eyes, there is a direct correlation between the eyes and liver function, which can be assessed diagnostically (jaundice, reddening of the eyes when drinking alcohol!).

K-N Gan Ki Mek begins at the inner nail tip of the little finger, extends along the palm of the hand to N 16, and continues in the palm of the hand to N 18, where it ends above the capitulum of MC IV.

Refresher: Important points of K-N Gan Ki Mek

- **N 1:** Source of liver energy, conditions of shock, nervousness

- **N 3:** Eye diseases, fatigue, sedates liver *yang*

- **N 5:** Together with N 18 and corresponding eye point on the middle finger as proven combination in all eye diseases, makes liver *qi* smooth

- **N 18:** Alarm point of the Liver Channel, for fatigue, all liver diseases

Korean Hand Acupuncture

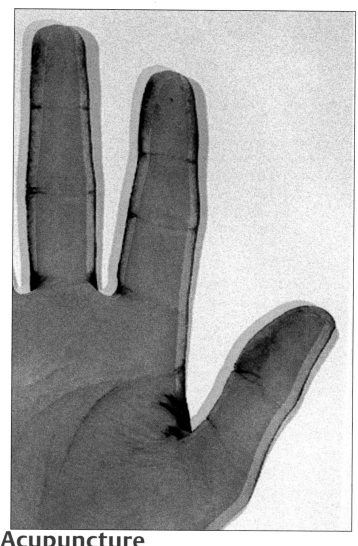

10 Chinese Hand Acupuncture

(H.-U. Hecker, A. Steveling, E.T. Peuker)

Introduction

Chinese hand acupuncture is a rarely used form of acupuncture that is often employed in combination with other acupuncture methods, for example, body and auricular acupuncture.

For the sake of completeness, it should be pointed out that a special school of hand acupuncture has developed in Korea which is increasingly being employed here in Europe as well.

In Western countries several hand acupuncture points have proved very effective and are also often used, for example, Point 1 (really two points) for the treatment of lumbago and ischialgia, or Point 14 for the treatment of throat–neck complaints.

Similar to the ear, scalp, and mouth, there is also a somatopic arrangement of various regions of the body in the area of the ventral and dorsal sides of the hand. By needling the corresponding acupuncture points, a regulatory effect can be exerted on these.

The disadvantage of hand acupuncture is the relatively painful nature of the treatment.

Technique

In hand acupuncture, acupuncture with lasers is more patient-friendly than the needle technique.

Treatment with the needle technique usually lasts 10–20 minutes and is therefore somewhat shorter than body acupuncture (approx. 30 minutes). Depending on the localization of the points, the needling depth may vary between 0.2 and 1 cm.

Good results are attributed to the use of electroacupuncture. Electrostimulation mainly uses frequencies of 3–10 Hz.

Needling of the palm of the hand can prove very difficult on account of the level of pain involved. Hardened skin in the palm area of the hand is also a problem.

When giving treatment via the points of the palm of the hand, laser acupuncture is the best option for patients who are very sensitive to pain.

Indications and Contraindications

The main indication is pain therapy.

There are no absolute contraindications. If individual points are extremely painful, they should be avoided.

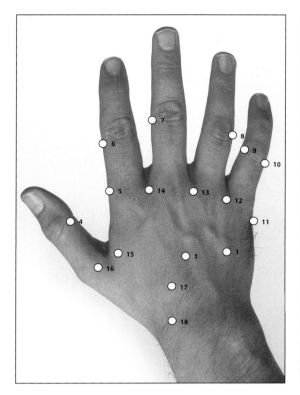

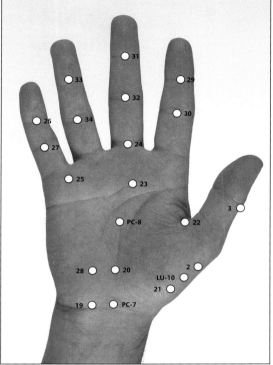

Hand acupuncture points on the dorsal surface of the hand

Hand acupuncture points on the palm of the hand

Hand Acupuncture Points on the Dorsal Surface of the Hand

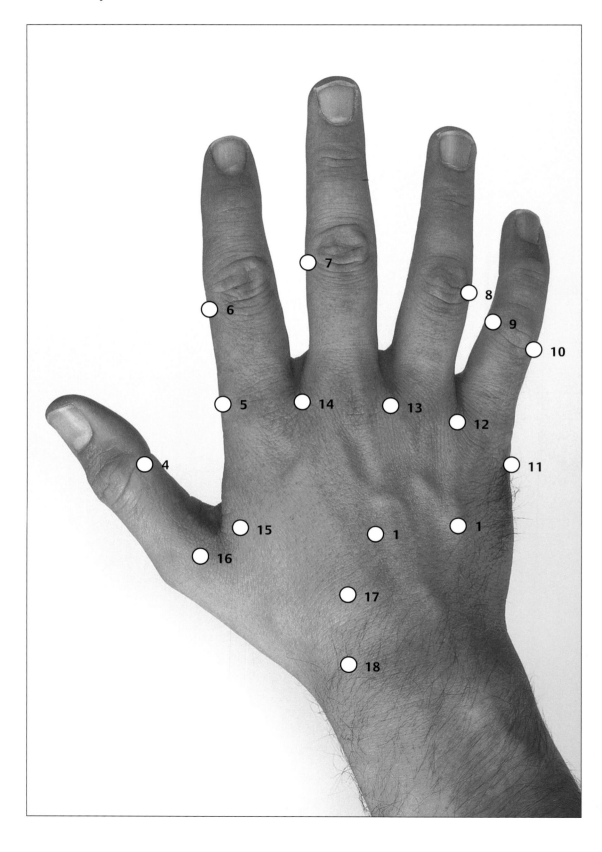

Hand Point 1 Lumbar Point, Leg Point

Location: There are two points in this connection which are each located at the proximal end of the metacarpal bone between fourth and fifth finger and second and third finger.

Indication: Lumboischialgia, Lumbar Vertebrae Zone (LVZ) syndrome.

As a rule, the points are needled jointly and firmly manipulated.

This is the most important point in Chinese hand acupuncture and is frequently used for acute LVZ syndrome or for lumboischialgia.

Both these points (there are two points) are needled using a sedative needle technique for acute complaints.

Hand Point 4 Eye Point

Location: On the ulnar side of the interphalangeal joint of the thumb, at the end of the flexion crease.

Indication: Complaints in the eye region.

Hand Point 5 Shoulder Point

Location: On the radial side of the metacarpophalangeal joint of the index finger, at the end of the flexion crease.

Indication: Shoulder–arm syndrome.

Hand Point 6 Forehead Point

Location: On the radial side of the proximal interphalangeal joint of the index finger, at the end of the flexion crease.

Indication: Cephalgia, sinusitis, and afflictions in the forehead–head region.

Hand Point 7 Parting Point

Location: On the radial side of the proximal interphalangeal joint of the index finger, at the end of the flexion crease.

Indication: Cephalgia, migraine.

Hand Point 8 Migraine Point, Half of the Head (on the right or left)

Location: On the ulnar side of the proximal interphalangeal joint of the fourth finger, at the end of the flexion crease.

Indication: Migraine, cephalgia, one-sided headache, and afflictions of the bile ducts and gallbladder.

Hand Point 9 Genital Point, Perineum Point

Location: On the radial side of the proximal interphalangeal joint of the little finger joint, at the end of the flexion crease.

Indication: Hemorrhoids, pain in the perineal region.

Hand Point 10 Back of the Head Point

Location: On the ulnar side of the proximal interphalangeal joint of the little finger joint, at the end of the flexion crease.

Indication: Occipital headache.

Hand Point 11 Spinal Column Point

Location: On the ulnar side of the base joint of the little finger, at the end of the flexion crease.

Indication: Spinal column syndrome, tinnitus, thoracodynia.

Chinese Hand Acupuncture

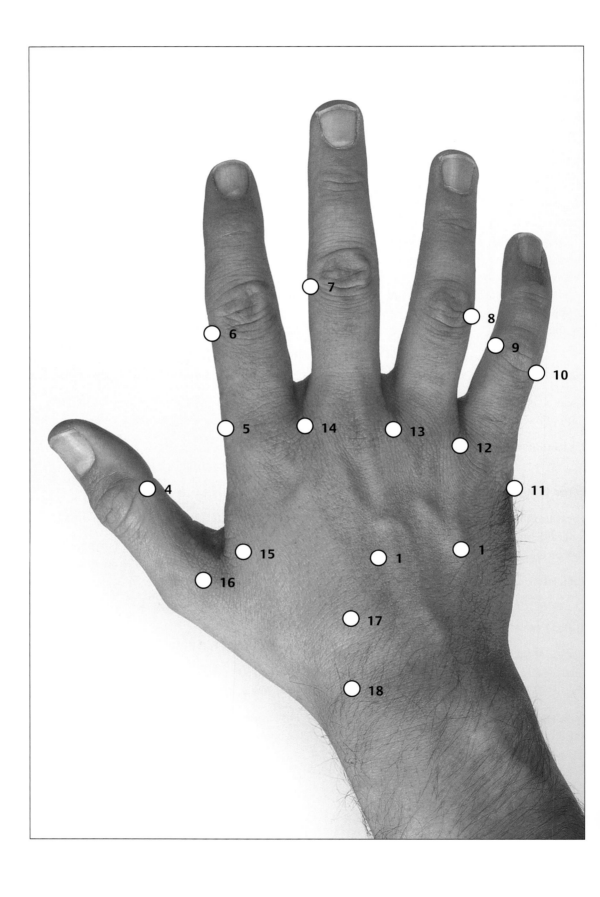

Hand Point 12   Sciatic Nerve Point

Location: On the ulnar side of the base joint of the ring finger.

Indication: Ischialgia, coxalgia, lumboischialgia.

Hand Point 13   Throat, Pharynx, and Larynx Point

Location: On the ulnar side of the base joint of the middle finger.

Indication: Laryngitis, pharyngitis, globus sensation, toothache.

Hand Point 14   Neck Point

Location: On the ulnar side of the base joint of the index finger.

Indication: Cervical vertebrae syndrome.

Besides Hand Point 1, Hand Point 14 is one of the most important points in hand acupuncture. Neck and back complaints can frequently be alleviated using a sedative needle technique.

Hand Point 15   Nosebleeds

Location: On the ulnar side of the edge of the web between thumb and index finger.

Indication: Nosebleeds.

Hand Point 16   Head

Location: On the ulnar side of the base joint of the thumb, at the end of the flexion crease.

Indication: Headaches.

Hand Point 17   Nose

Location: Dorsal side of hand in the angle formed by metacarpal bones 1 and 2.

Indication: Rhinitis, sinusitis.

Hand Point 18   Wrist Point

Location: In the flexion crease of the wrist approx. 1/2 *cun* ulnar of the anatomical snuffbox.

Indication: Afflictions of the wrist. Hand acupuncture points on the dorsal surface of the hand.

For comparison: The hand acupuncture points on the palm of the hand

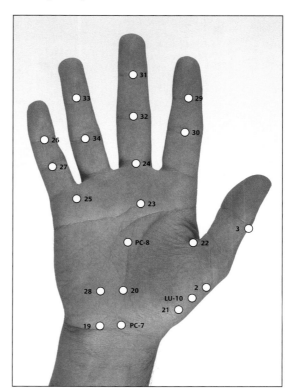

Chinese Hand Acupuncture

Hand Acupuncture Points on the Palm of the Hand

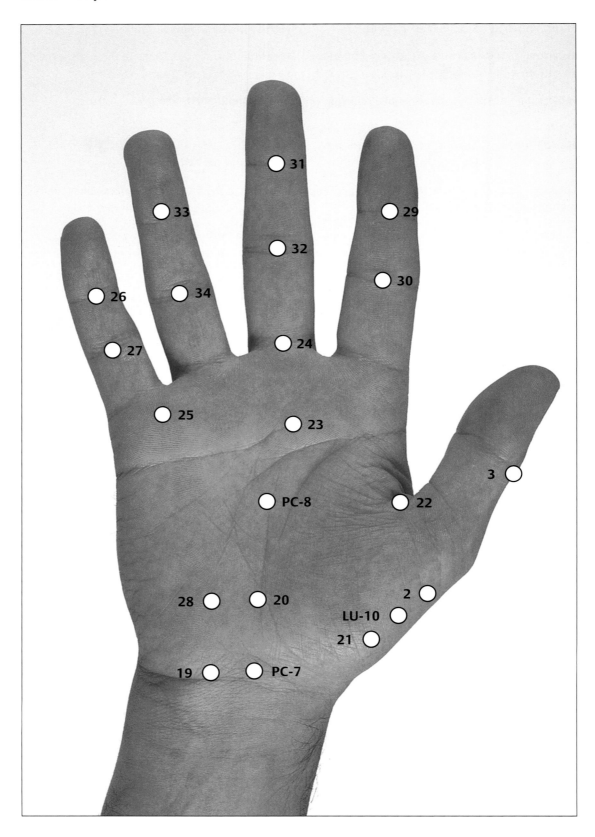

Hand Point 2   Ankle Point, Foot Point

Location: On the radial side of the base joint of the thumb, at the end of the flexion crease.

Indication: Joint pain in the region of the foot.

Hand Point 3   Chest Point, Thorax Point

Location: On the radial side of the interphalangeal joint of the thumb, at the end of the flexion crease.

Indication: Thoracodynia, intercostal neuralgia.

Hand Point 19   Upper Abdomen

Location: Somewhat ulnar of the PC-7 on the lower edge of the palm of the hand.

Indication: Upper abdominal pain.

Hand Point 20   Foot Joint

Location: Approx. 1 *cun* proximal to PC-8 in the palm of the hand.

Indication: Pain in the foot joint.

Hand Point 21   Colds

Location: Somewhat below and ulnar to LU-10 on the ball of the thumb.

Indication: Colds.

Hand Point 22   Hysteria

Location: With the thumb abducted in the center of the web of the thumb and index finger in the palm of the hand.

Indication: Hysteria.

Hand Point 23   Bronchitis

Location: Approx. 1 *cun* proximal to the web of the second and third finger in the palm of the hand.

Indication: Bronchitis.

Hand Point 24   Mouth

Location: In the middle of the metacarpophalangeal joint of the third finger in the palm of the hand.

Indication: Stomatitis.

Hand Point 25   Heart

Location: Approx. 1/2 *cun* proximal to the web between fourth and fifth finger in the palm of the hand.

Indication: Functional heart complaints.

Hand Point 26   Kidney

Location: In the middle of the distal interphalangeal joint of the fifth finger in the palm of the hand.

Indication: Kidney diseases (pain).

Hand Point 27   Enuresis

Location: In the middle of the proximal interphalangeal joint of the fifth finger in the palm of the hand.

Indication: Enuresis.

Hand Point 28   Sweating

Location: 1 *cun* above Point 19 in the palm of the hand.

Indication: Hyperhidrosis.

Chinese Hand Acupuncture

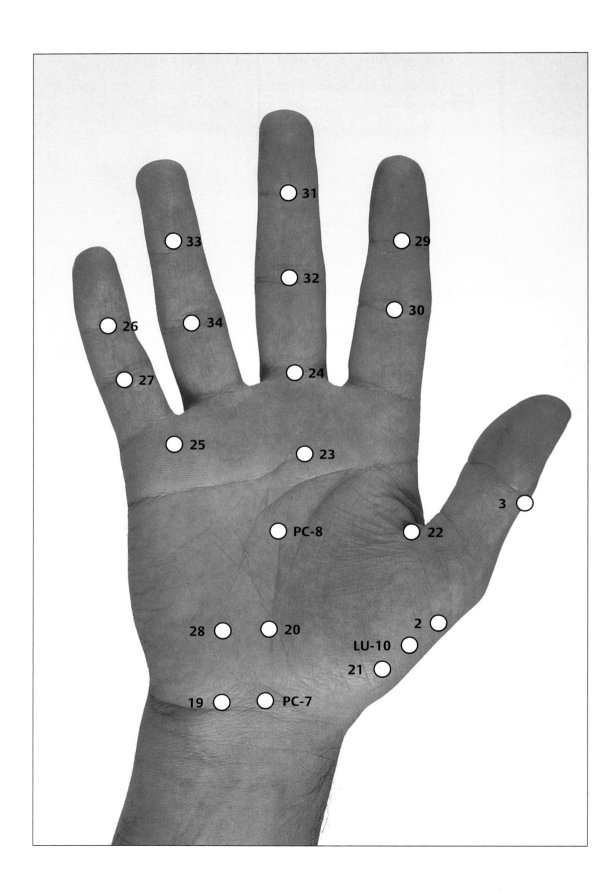

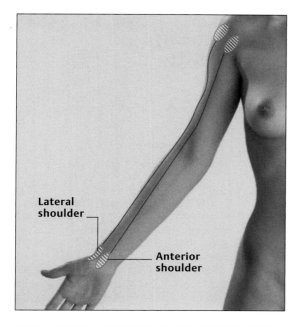

Lateral shoulder

Anterior shoulder

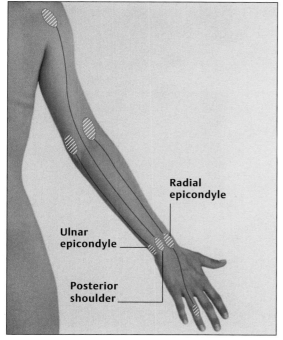

Radial epicondyle

Ulnar epicondyle

Posterior shoulder

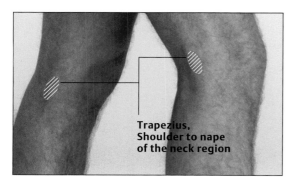

Trapezius, Shoulder to nape of the neck region

Projection Zones of the Shoulder and Elbow According to *Siener*

Similar to acupuncture, areas specific to the Small Intestine, Triple Burner, and Large Intestine or Lung Channel surrounding the wrist joint are used for the dorsal, lateral, and anterior shoulder. An extension of the "response ray" in a distal direction surrounding the finger joints may also be effective here.

The lateral epicondyle of the humerus is located in the region of the styloid process of the ulna and the medial epicondyle of the humerus in the region of the styloid process of the radius. A particularly effective site for radial epicondylopathy is located in the region of the articular capsule of the proximal and distal interphalangeal joint of the fourth finger (both lateral and medial). It should be remembered that, in accordance with the axis principles of acupuncture, treatment should begin on the foot in the case of neck, shoulder, and arm complaints (just as according to *Mann*, LR-3 can be the most effective point for cervical syndrome).

This is further reinforced according to manual treatment principles, as a relatively large number of cervical and cervicogenic complaints (shoulder and elbow) are the result of an imbalance in the lower extremity and the pelvis with subsequent compensatory scoliosis. According to the principles of craniosacral osteopathy, there are no isolated upper or lower imbalances so that the common principle of top-to-bottom coupling in acupuncture is also plausible.

Where the hamstrings are attached to the fibula there is an effective zone for relaxation of the upper trapezius.

Both *Matsumoto* and *Mann* indicate the effectiveness of the region surrounding SP-9 in the trapezius area in some cases.

NPPOT

Areas for the Treatment of Internal Organs

Different rules apply to the topography of the internal organs, and the pattern resembles a somatotopy; the head is represented on the knee and the face on the patella. The cranial tibial area and the adjacent musculature correspond to the thorax organs and the central lower leg region to the upper and lower abdominal organs.

The projection zones can be located either according to this large, graphic principle or by using the "very point" dabbing technique. However, this is not a precise means of determining whether the point located corresponds to the region to be treated or rather indicates another active point.

The face is represented on the patella with the bridge of the nose at the 12 o'clock position (bilaterally), the eyes at around the 2 o'clock position on the left knee and the 10 o'clock position on the right knee. The temporomandibular joint is located on the edge of the right patella at the 9 o'clock position and on the left edge at the 3 o'clock position. The tonsils are located at the edge of the right patella at the 7 to 8 o'clock position and at the edge of the left patella at the 4 to 5 o'clock position.

The epiglottis is located on the lower edge of the patella at the 6 o'clock position, bilaterally, while the trachea, thyroid gland, and bronchial tubes follow in a caudal direction.

The internal organs of the left and right halves of the body are located on the left or right lower leg respectively. The liver is on the right lower leg and the spleen is on the left lower leg. The mammary gland is on the lower leg in the region of the Stomach Channel, which also represents a direct top-to-bottom projection.

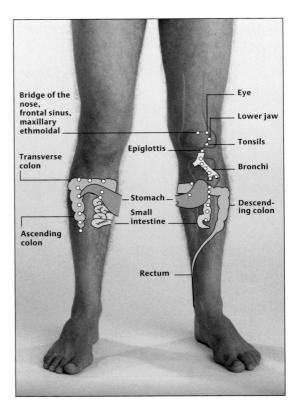

Bridge of the nose, frontal sinus, maxillary ethmoidal

Transverse colon

Ascending colon

Epiglottis

Stomach

Small intestine

Rectum

Eye

Lower jaw

Tonsils

Bronchi

Descending colon

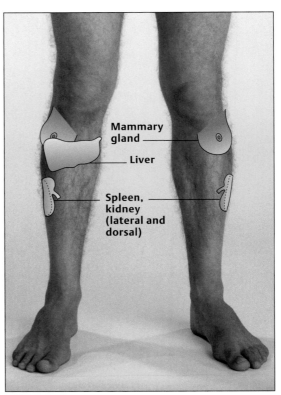

Mammary gland

Liver

Spleen, kidney (lateral and dorsal)

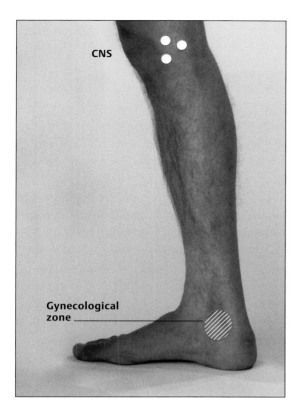

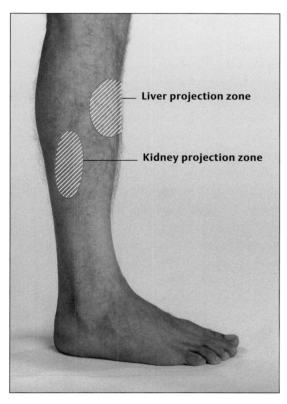

The internal genitals and gynecological regions are typically found within the Kidney Channel at KI-4 to KI-6.

Using the "very point technique" within the medial knee area, an equilateral triangle can also be found, which has a hormonal and psychotropic regulatory effect. These points represent the Hypothalamus, Pituitary Gland, and Limbic System.

Treatment Technique

The effective points can be found by means of trial and error and the "very point" technique using an acupuncture needle or size 20 cannula with a 5 ml procaine syringe. However, the points can also be found using auriculocardiac reflex (ACR) or Applied Kinesiology therapy localization.

The author's experience to date suggests an acupuncture needle is more effective in the treatment of internal organs, where needling is in the muscular region. However, an injection of 0.2 ml procaine surrounding the locomotor system points is more favourable where periosteal treatment is the most effective. However, an acupuncture needle can also be used here, as accuracy is paramount.

Sensitive patients may find this treatment technique very painful and be unable to tolerate it. In this case, electric point searching with a resistance meter can be used (standard acupoint searching devices) followed by laser treatment.

The author rates the pulsed laser (Nextlaser), made by Sedatelec. This device may produce *qi*-like sensations during radiation treatment. There are also some competitively priced laser pointers used in slide presentations, which may also be effective.

In the case of diseases of the locomotor system, there is an immediate effect, as with auricular or scalp acupuncture, if the correct point is treated. The effect usually lasts longer per treatment than with scalp acupuncture according to *Yamamoto*.

The technique can, of course, be supplemented by needling and therapeutic local anesthesia of the painful sites (e.g. the sacroiliac joint) and the local trigger points, as well as by Manual Therapy, and can therefore be more effective as a result.

Indications

Locomotor System

In diseases of the locomotor system, the result is similar to that following treatment by a different microsystem. If successful, results are immediately apparent. If not, a different system must be used (scalp acupuncture, auricular acupuncture, body acupuncture, etc.).

This method is recommended for the following: lumbar syndrome, lumbar-like complaints, sacroiliac joint syndrome, coxalgia, coxarthrosis, gonalgia, gonarthrosis, pain in the ankle joint, Cervical Vertebrae Zone (CVZ) syndrome, shoulder–arm syndrome, epicondylopathy, pain in the wrist joint, cephalgia, and, in particular, tension headaches.

Some diagnoses are rather vague, for example, "lumbar-like complaints." This is, however, not critical, as in the case of both radicular and pseudoradicular syndromes, an effect may be achieved without considering the etiology.

Organ Diseases

Treatment may be effective for sinusitides, bronchitides and functional disturbances of the thyroid gland including nodular goiter, where the thyroid hormone levels can become normalized.

Indications also include gastrointestinal disturbances such as gastritis, gastralgia, Crohn disease and ulcerative colitis.

Complaints of the kidneys and deferent urinary passages and dysmenorrhea may be treated with this method and, in addition, mastopathies. Surprisingly, an improvement of the tissue structure can also be achieved here by treating the mammary gland area, which is usually in the region of the Stomach Channel.

Hormonal imbalances are treated via the "central nervous system (CNS) triangle", made up of the hypothalamus, pituitary gland, and limbic system. This combination also has a psychotropic effect.

Treatment Areas of Muscular Disturbances and Vertebral Lesions

Treatment Areas of Muscular Disturbances

Where there is muscle dysfunction, local reflex zones and trigger points that can be clearly assigned to a channel (cf. tables p. 308 onwards), can be palpated. For example, the anterior tibial muscle has typical and frequent reflex zones that correspond to points ST-36 and ST-38, resulting in the assignment of this muscle to the Stomach Channel.

The distal acupuncture point most likely to be effective in treating individual muscle dysfunctions can be found as a result of this assignment, as the acupuncture channels correspond to the sequence of the trigger points and reflex zones in the muscles of a kinetic chain. Remote points are no more than particularly effective points in the periphery of a muscular lesion chain that are all found in the region of the wrist, ankle joint or knee.

Individual muscles can also be treated using this method. The cutaneous segment, where the muscle lies, is first located and then assigned to a typical point on the channel, belonging to the segment (cf. tables p. 312 onwards) near the wrist joint, ankle joint, or knee joint. Consequently, this corresponds to the simple method indicated by *Siener*, who at the time spoke about having to drop a perpendicular from the painful region, from the proximal painful area to the periphery and finding a point of maximum response on the large joints.

Where corresponding acupuncture points are listed in the tables on page 308 et seq., this refers to an area in which the point of maximum response and maximum effect can be found (e.g. by means of a "dabbing" needle using the "very point" technique).

It is recommended that muscular and bony areas in this peripheral region be examined, as a needle (or laser) in the muscle can from time to time have a completely different effect to stimulation of the periosteum.

It should be remembered that the local points in the musculature must also be treated.

Treatment Areas of Vertebral Lesions

The same method of segmental organization and overlapping of dermatome, myotome, and sclerotome can be used to treat vertebral lesions (vertebral dysfunctions or subluxations).

The simplest options for segment-related acupuncture of vertebral lesions are listed in the following illustrations and tables. These can be used on their own or as a supplement to Manual Therapy.

Muscles, Their Local Reflex Zones and Effective Remote Points: Cervical Segments

Muscle	Muscular local points	Best remote points
Sternocleidomastoid muscle	TB-16, LI-18, ST-10	TB-5, GB-41
Scalene muscle	LI-17, LI-18, SI-16	SI-4, TB-5, SI-3
Superior trapezius muscle	TB-15	TB-5; BL-38, BL-39
Medial trapezius muscle	BL-13, BL-14	BL-38, BL-39
Inferior trapezius muscle	BL-16, BL-17	BL-59
Levator muscle of scapula	SI-15	SI-3
Subclavius muscle	ST-13	ST-38
Greater pectoral muscle	ST-15, ST-16; SP-19, SP-20	ST-38, SP-9
Smaller pectoral muscle	ST-15, ST-16	ST-38
Smaller and greater rhomboid muscles	BL-12, BL-13	SI-3/BL-62
Supraspinatus muscle	SI-12	SI-3/BL-62
Infraspinatus muscle	SI-11	SI-3
Anterior serratus muscle	SP-21	SP-9
Subscapular muscle	SI-12	SI-3
Teres major muscle	SI-9	SI-3
Latissimus dorsi muscle	Point outside of the channels, circa EX-129 (*Hou Ye*)	
Teres minor muscle	SI-9	SI-3
Deltoid muscle	LI-15, TB-14, SI-10	ST-38
Biceps brachii muscle	LU-4, (PC-4)	LU-7
Coracobrachialis muscle	LU-1	LU-7
Brachialis muscle	HT-2, LU-3, LU-4	SI-3
Triceps brachii muscle	TB-12, TB-13	TB-5
Brachioradialis muscle	LI-10, LI-12	LI-4
Extensor carpi radius longus muscle	LI-10	LI-4
Extensor carpi radius brevis muscle	LI-9	LI-4
Supinator muscle	LU-6	LU-7

Muscle	Muscular local points	Best remote points
Extensor digitorum muscle	TB-9	TB-5
Etensor carpi ulnaris muscle	TB-9	SI-6
Abductor pollicus longus muscle	LI-6, 7	SI-4
Extensor pollicis brevis muscle	LI-6, 7	SI-4
Extensor pollicis longus muscle	TB-5	SI-4, *Louzhen*
Extensor indicis muscle	TB-5	SI-4, *Louzhen*
Pronator teres muscle	PC-8	PE-6
Flexor carpi radius muscle	PC-4	LU-7, PC-6
Palmaris longus muscle	PC-4	PC-6
Flexor digitorum superficialis muscle	PC-4, SI-7	LU-7, PC-6/SI-3, HT-8
Flexor digitorum profundus muscle (first to third finger)	PC-4	PC-6
Flexor digitorum profundus muscle (fourth to fifth finger)	SI-7	SI-3
Flexor pollicis longus muscle	LU-6	LU-7
Pronator quadratus muscle	PE-5	PC-6
Abductor pollicis brevis muscle	LU-10	LU-10
Opponens pollicis muscle	LU-10	LU-10
Flexor pollicis brevis muscle	LU-10	LU-10
Pollicis adductor muscle	LU-10	LU-10
Lumbricalis muscles 1 to 3	PC-8	PC-8
Flexor carpi ulnaris muscle	SI-7	SI-3
Opponens digitarum minimus muscle	SI-3	SI-3

NPPOT

Muscles, Their Local Reflex Zones and Effective Remote Points: Thoracic, Lumbar, and Sacral

Muscle	Muscular local points	Best remote points
Erector spinae muscle	Bladder Channel	BL-62, SI-3
Rectus abdominus muscle	KI-11 to KI-21	CV-2
Oblique extensor abductor muscle	SP-14, SP-15; GB-26	GB-41
Oblique internal abdominus muscle	SP-14, SP-15; GB-26	GB-41
Quadratus lumborum muscle	BL-20 to BL-25, BL-50 to BL-52	BL-59
Psoas muscle	ST-"30.5", LR-11	SP-9
Iliacus muscle	GB-27, ST-"30.5", LR-11	GB-41, SP-9
Sartorius muscle	SP-11	SP-9
Quadriceps femoris muscle	ST-32	ST-41
Adductor brevis and longus muscles	LR-9	KI-3
Gracilis muscle	LR-9	KI-3
Adductor magnus muscle	LR-9	KI-3, unnumbered points on the Kidney Channel
Gluteus medius muscle	GB-29, GB-30	GB-38
Tensor fasciae latae muscle	GB-29	GB-38
Gluteus maximus muscle	BL-53, BL-54; GB-30	GB-38
Piriformis muscle	BL-54	BL-60
Hip external rotators (gemelli muscle, obturatorius internal muscle, quadratus femoris muscle)	GB-30	GB-39, BL-60
Biceps femoris muscle	BL-37, BL-60	
Semimembranosus muscle, semitendinosus muscle	Unnumbered points on the Kidney Channel	KI-3
Tibialis anterior muscle	ST-36, ST-38	ST-41
Extensor hallucis longus muscle, extensor digitorum longus muscle	ST-39	ST-41

Muscle	Muscular local points	Best remote points
Peroneus longus muscle, peroneus brevis muscle, peroneus tertius muscle	GB-38 to GB-40	GB-41
Gastrocnemius muscle	BL-55 to BL-57	BL-60
Popliteus muscle	BL-56	BL-60
Soleus muscle	BL-57 to BL-59	BL-60
Tibialis posterior muscle	BL-5, BL-58	BL-60
Flexor hallucis longus muscle	KI-7	KI-2
Flexor hallucis brevis muscle	KI-2	KI-2

NPPOT

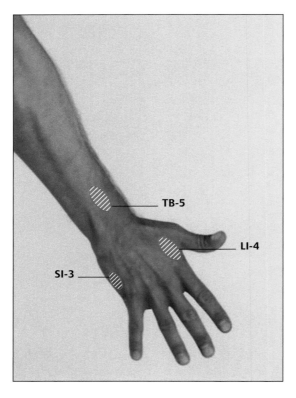

Segment-related acupuncture: C1 to C4

Segment-related acupuncture: C5

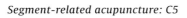

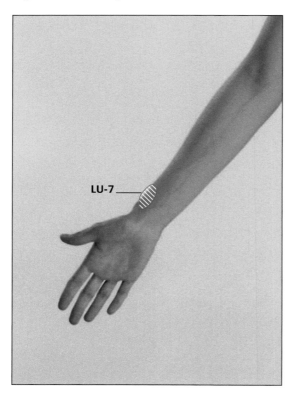

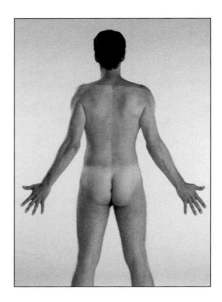

Segments C1 to C4

Cervical segments	Points
C1 to C4	TB-5, SI-3, LI-4
C5	LU-7, LI-4

Segment C5

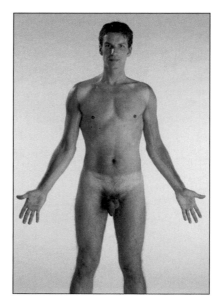

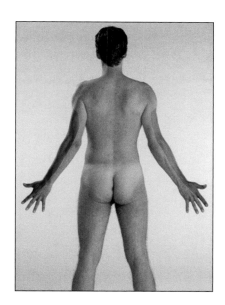

Segment C6

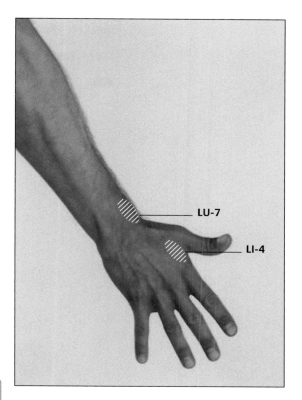

Segment-related acupuncture: C6

Cervical segments	Points
C6	LU-7, LI-4
C7	PC-6, TB-5

Segment-related acupuncture: C7

Segment C7

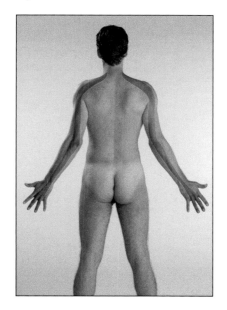

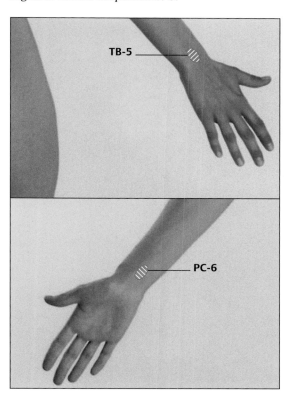

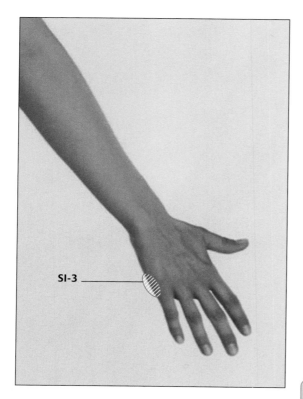

Segment-related acupuncture: C8

Segment-related acupuncture: T1

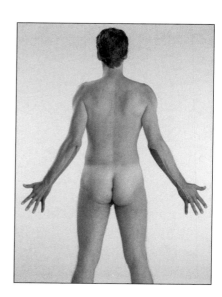

Segment C8

Cervical segments	Points
C8	SI-3
T1	HT-8, SI-3

Segment T1

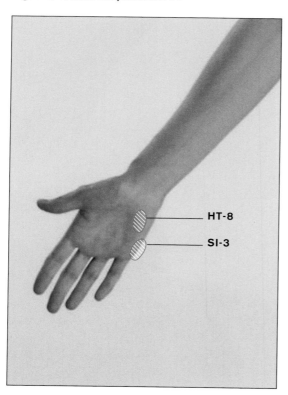

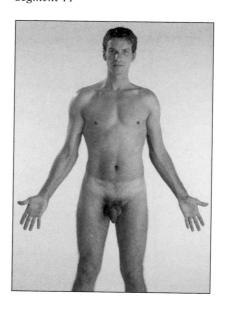

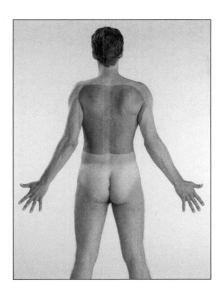

Segments T2 to T12

Thoracic segments	Points
T2 to T12	TB-5 and GB-40
	TB-8 and GB-41
	SI-3 and BL-62
	Hua Tuo's paravertebral points
Lumbar segments	**Points**
L1/2	LR-3

Segments L1/2

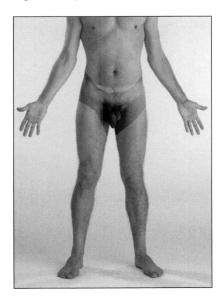

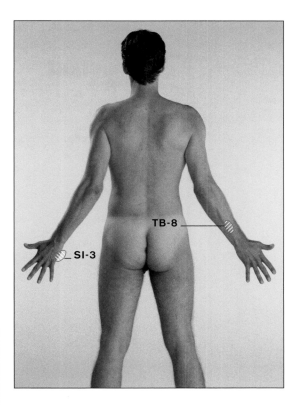

Segment-related acupuncture: T2 to T12

Segment-related acupuncture: L1/2

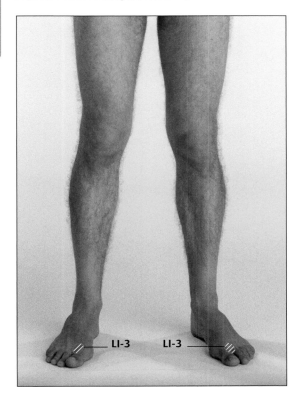

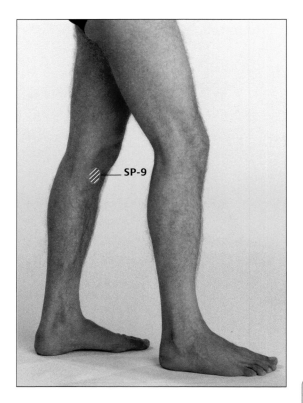

Segment-related acupuncture: L3

Segment-related acupuncture: L4

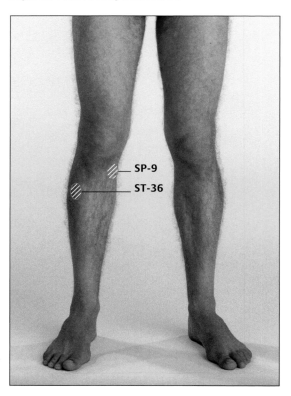

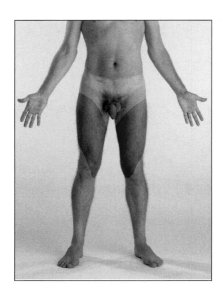

Segment L3.

Lumbar segments	Points
L3	SP-9
L4	SP-9, ST-36

Segment L4

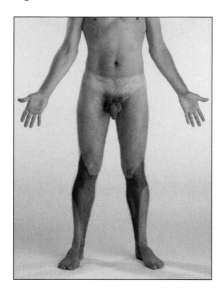

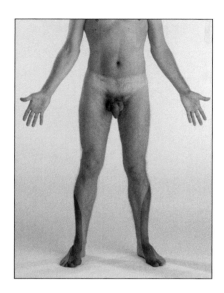

Segment L5

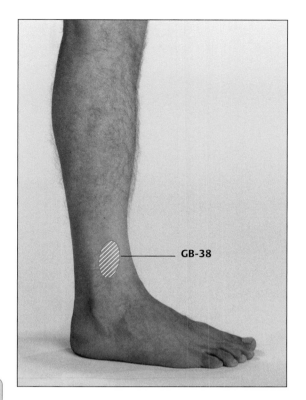

Segment-related acupuncture: L5

Lumbar segments	Points
L5	GB-38
S1	KI-3, BL-60

Segment-related acupuncture: S1

Segment S1

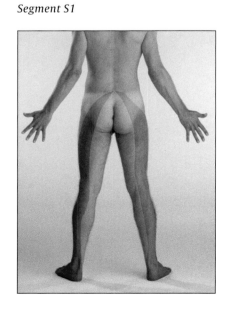

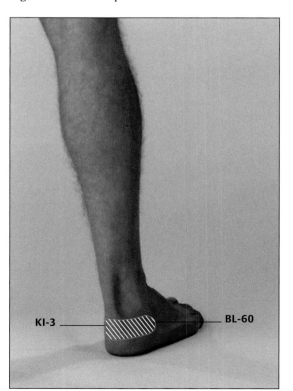

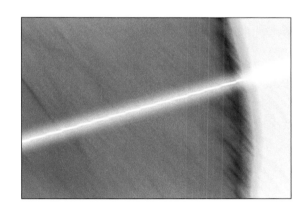

12 Laser Therapy

(M. Wiesner-Zechmeister)

Use of Low-Level Laser in Fractal Microsystems

One of the greatest innovations of recent decades in acupuncture has been the use of laser. The acupuncture point or area to be stimulated is influenced by an electromagnetic impulse, the laser light. This gives the acupuncturist a "light needle" which makes it possible to find the indication for acupuncture significantly more often, for example, in children, and to considerably increase the treatment options open to the acupuncturist. At the same time, scientists began to take an interest in the phenomenon that makes it possible to stimulate and influence biologically active points with a special light. The results of the various studies represent an enormous enrichment of research into acupuncture. The word "laser" is an acronym for "light amplification by stimulated emission of radiation."

Einstein discovered the laser principle shortly after the turn of the 20th century. However, it was not until the 1960's that the first laser, a ruby laser, was manufactured. Shortly afterwards the first helium–neon laser was developed. This emits a red light with a wavelength of 632.8 nanometers.

The Functional Principle of the Helium–Neon Laser

A laser tube contains a mixture of helium and neon gas. A voltage is applied to this mixture, dispatching the electrons of the helium atoms on a higher-energy, metastable path. By colliding with the neon atoms, the electrons return to their original path. The energy arising in this way is released in the form of light quanta, so-called photons. The light is polarized between the cavity mirrors while one of the mirrors from which the laser beam emerges is semipermeable.

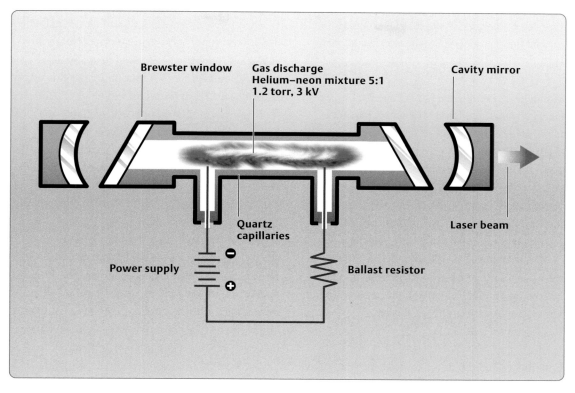

The functional principle of the helium–neon laser

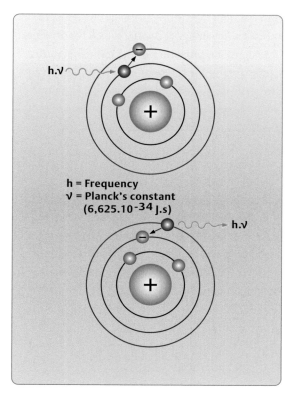

h = Frequency
ν = Planck's constant
(6,625.10^{-34} J.s)

The atomic model

The Laser Light

Properties

Two key properties distinguish laser light from normal light, namely monochromasy and coherence.

Monochromasy: Visible light is a small part of electromagnetic radiation, which also includes many other familiar kinds of radiation such as, for example, UV radiation or radio waves besides light. What we recognize as light consists of different colors of the spectrum ranging from violet to red. Visible wavelengths oscillate between approx. 350 and 700 nanometers. The range above 700 nanometers is known as the infrared range.

Monochromatic laser light only comprises a single wavelength. The light which is emitted by a helium–neon tube is, for example, a pure red light with a single wavelength, in this case 632.8 nanometers.

Coherence: Coherence means that there is a fixed phase relationship between all components of laser radiation—it is therefore an extremely highly ordered light. According to studies by *Popp*, the transparency of living tissues, which represent a very dense material for normal light, is significantly greater for coherent laser light. American scientists demonstrated that weak laser light is not, as expected, reflected on the surface of radiated plant roots but penetrates practically the whole root loss-free.

The view today is that a continuous rather than a pulsed beam should be used. This ensures the continuous emission of electromagnetic stimulation. Frequencies like those achieved by "chopping up a laser beam" bear no relevance to treatment at present. In this regard, it has not been possible to verify the therapeutic effect of frequencies used by *Bahr* and *Nogier* to date.

Depth of Penetration

According to the Monte Carlo definition, the penetration depth of a beam is defined as the depth at which a third of the original beam is still evident. 10^{17} photons per second are released from a 10-mW laser. With the lasers used in acupuncture, the penetration depth is 2–4 mm, so that at this depth approx. 3×10^{16} photons are still evident. Thereafter, sufficient photons are still available at a depth of several centimeters, ensuring biological induction. When the laser is used to stimulate the acupuncture zones of fractal microsystems, the depth of penetration plays a more subordinate role, as these zones are situated only a few millimeters under the skin.

The view today is that the following are crucial for the special effect of laser light compared with normal light: monochromasy permits the application of a high power density of a quite specific wavelength at the acupuncture point in spite of the seemingly low output of the low-level laser in the milliwatt range. Coherence seems to be responsible for the significantly greater depth of penetration of laser light into the tissues compared with normal light, while electromagnetic induction of tissue radiation immediately under the skin is still being debated.

How Does Laser Work in Acupuncture?

The elementary processes which enable organic life in the first place occur at an atomic and sub-atomic level. These processes alone make it possible for organic structures to be formed and to interact. They form the basis of every biochemical process. The laws of quantum physics apply at this level and electromagnetism dominates as a major force. All organic structures are in permanent interaction and all organic structures emit coherent, electromagnetic waves. This electromagnetic radiation is the most elementary form of mutual exertion of influence and information transfer of biological systems.

Biological systems are open systems, i.e. they are accessible to the exertion of influence from outside and pass on altered information each time according to the corresponding influence.

This passing on of electromagnetic information may be the explanation for the remote influence of acupuncture points and also explains why there is no anatomical substrate for the transfer of information.

Electromagnetic waves are released with increased frequency at the synapses of nerves. As a result of interaction with other nerve fibers and their waves, oscillations may interfere and thus form interference patterns similar to holograms. From a biophysical perspective, these interference points correspond to acupuncture points which may contain information about the operation of large parts of the body. As biophysical coordinating points, these acupuncture points are naturally accessible to the exertion of influence from outside, whether they correspond to classical acupuncture points or fractal microsystems. The traditional means is mechanical irritation with a needle. Laser stimulation represents an additional, very elegant, direct, electromagnetic influence. The release of photons induced in this way at the acupuncture point may boost existing, weak radiation.

The Practical Application of Laser

In contrast to surgical lasers, which all operate in watts and are used as light scalpels, lasers which operate in milliwatts are used in acupuncture. They are performance class III, mainly performance class IIIb, and are therefore subject to radiation protection provisions.

These lasers do not heat up the tissues at all and their sole purpose is biostimulation. In accordance with the current level of knowledge, lasers with an output of between 6 and 15 mW (the ratings always relate to 1 cm^2) are usually used. With the exception of oral acupuncture, the tip of the laser is placed directly on the corresponding area and the duration of radiation is between 10 and 15 seconds. Lasers emitting a constant beam are used.

Frequencies like those resulting from "chopping up" the constant beam are not used here.

As many studies show, the biological, biochemical, and biophysical responses of the organism can above all be traced back to the wavelength of laser light used. The desired effects can be achieved in acupuncture by lasers emitting a light in the red light or in the adjacent infrared light range. For empirical and practical reasons, as well as on account of various studies, a red light laser is currently to be recommended.

Particularly when used in various special forms of acupuncture, laser has a number of advantages. As the zones are located immediately below the skin, the laser can stimulate them without any difficulty.

In patients who are very sensitive to pain or who would be loath to agree to needle acupuncture, such as children, for example, laser acupuncture can be carried out at any time as it is practically pain-free. A combination of laser acupuncture and needle acupuncture is quite possible.

Although the areas used for various fractal microsystems are exactly defined, the zones to be treated in each case must be precisely located on an individual basis. These corresponding zones are characterized by increased sensitivity to pressure pain and by changes in the consistency of the underlying tissue compared with the surrounding area and frequently by changes in the surface as well. This results in the increased conductivity of the skin—the resistance of the skin is reduced. Measurement of skin resistance is integrated into many laser devices, providing valuable assistance in finding the respective zone for treatment. However, it should be pointed out that the measuring of skin resistance cannot in any way replace the testing of pressure pain and tissue consistency.

Microsystems and System Theory

Until now, there was no explanation for the existence of microsystems in anatomy. It was system theory, which sees the construction of organic structures in a completely different light and reinterprets the interaction of the organism with the environment, which provided the explanation for microsystems.

System theory views an organism as a self-regulating, open system that is in permanent interaction with the environment, constantly absorbing information and energy from the environment, processing this, and passing it on again in another form. The organism is in a permanent equilibrium of flow, the physiological processes are irreversible, and their chief purpose is that of self-regulation.

From the perspective of system theory, the structure of the organism is fractal. The fractal structure of nature is currently causing a sensational revolution throughout the entire scientific world.

Fractal structures reflect the overall structure in every detail. They are found throughout nature—man has a fractal structure, too. Many anatomical structures such as the lung, the kidney, or the intestine have been recognized as fractal, i.e., they have a structure which reflects the whole. Individual microsystems are also an obvious indication of the fractal structure of the organism. Corresponding areas for the whole organism are found—arranged accordingly—at various locations on the surface of the body or the immediately underlying structures. A very obvious example of this is the ear in which the whole organism is reflected as an inverted embryo. It is interesting that the topical assignment of various parts of the body is not only achieved in the individual microsystems but that the Chinese organ systems are also reflected in various microsystems, as shown by the Y-points in *Yamamoto* scalp acupuncture.

Happily, experience shows that individual, fractal microsystems can be linked to diagnostic treatment concepts.

Thus, it is usually quite possible to also treat changes, for example, those detected in an organ system in abdominal wall diagnosis according to *Yamamoto*, via the ear or via the zones of Korean hand acupuncture.

This new, holistic way of looking at things will reveal completely new diagnostic and therapeutic possibilities in the future.

Applications of Laser Acupuncture

Application in Auricular Acupuncture

The use of laser has proved its worth for many years in auricular acupuncture. After precise localization of the area concerned, this is stimulated by direct application of the tip of the laser for 10–15 seconds. Frequently, a sensation of warmth in the sense of a *de qi* sensation is felt. Unlike stimulation with a needle, use of the laser naturally involves no risk of perichondritis.

Use in combination with traditional body acupuncture or microsystem areas is quite possible.

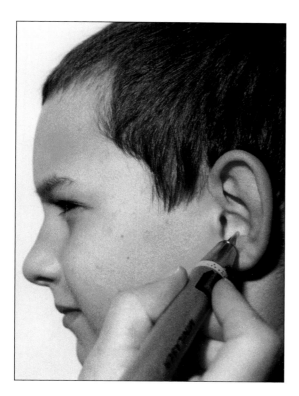

Stimulation of Auricular Point 101 (Lung)

Application in Scalp Acupuncture
According to *Yamamoto*

Here, too, the laser can be used without any difficulty on Zones A–H and on the Y-points. The
tremendous efficacy of laser stimulation is demonstrated precisely in the case of scalp acupuncture.
A disadvantage is that a *de qi* sensation cannot be
triggered as frequently as with needle stimulation,
making prior, precise localization of the point a
fundamental prerequisite. The *de qi* sensation,
insofar as it can be triggered, is usually experienced as a sensation of warmth. Here, too, the
laser is applied directly to the area. The duration of
radiation varies from 10–30 seconds.

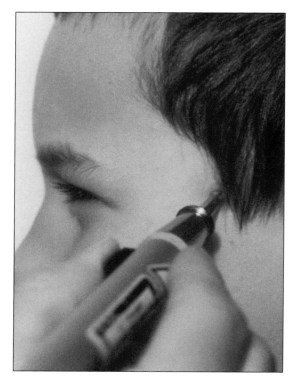

Stimulation of the Kidney Zone
according to Yamamoto

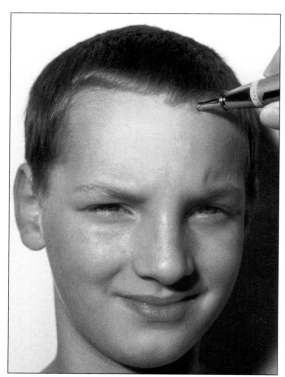

Stimulation of a point in Zone B
according to Yamamoto

Application in Oral Acupuncture According to *Gleditsch*

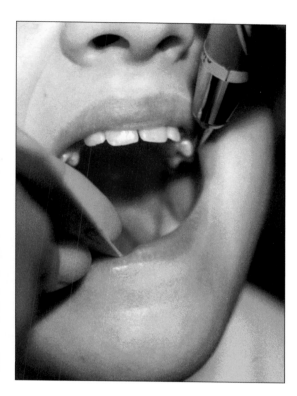

Laser stimulation in oral acupuncture

The traditional stimulation of areas in oral acupuncture takes place by means of injection of a local anesthetic. Stimulation of the corresponding zones by laser represents the only meaningful and practicable alternative with equivalent efficacy. Here it is usually not possible and advisable to apply the tip of the laser directly to the area concerned. In order to find the area concerned from a distance of several centimeters, it is necessary to use a laser which emits a correspondingly bundled beam. Simply for practical reasons it is also recommended that a red light laser be used here, as the area on which the laser beam has an effect can be precisely located. This is not possible with an infrared laser.

Here, too, the duration of radiation is usually between 10–20 seconds per area. Due to strong reflection by the mucous membranes, the therapist must always wear protective glasses.

Laser Therapy

Application in Korean Hand Acupuncture

Experience in using laser in Korean hand acupuncture is still relatively new. However, the treatment of diseases of the locomotor system via Korean hand acupuncture points using direct stimulation with a red light laser has proved highly effective. Here, too, the duration of radiation is between 10–30 seconds.

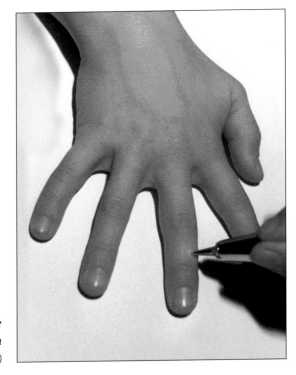

Korean hand acupuncture: Stimulation of a zone of the Bladder Channel in the region of the Cervical Vertebrae Zone (approx. L5/6)

Application in New Point-Based Pain and Organ Therapy (NPPOT)

Here, too, laser application is successful although spontaneous treatment success like that obtained traditionally by injecting a local anesthetic into the corresponding zone is not so obvious. In chronic diseases, however, which usually require several treatments, the application of laser has proved its worth both in monotherapy and in combination with traditional forms of acupuncture. The duration of radiation of individual zones is approx. 10–30 seconds.

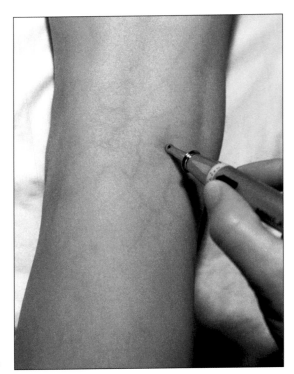

Laser stimulation in the region of the projection of the shoulder

13 Appendix

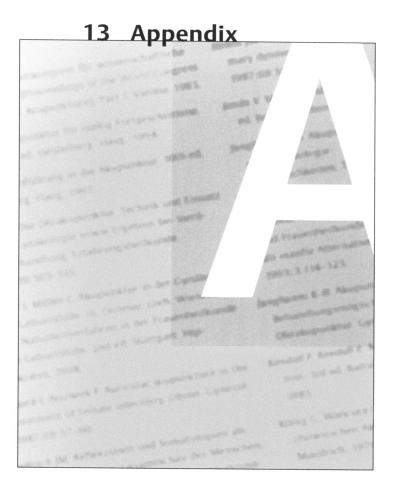

Further Reading

Bahr FR. Einführung in die wissenschaftliche Akupunkur. 6th ed. Braunschweig: Vieweg; 1995.

Bahr FR, Reis A, Straube EM, Strittmatter B, Suwanda S. Skriptum für die Aufbaustufe aller Akupunkturverfahren. 4th ed. Munich: Deutsche Akademie für Akupunktur & Aurikulomedizin e.V.; 1993.

Bergsmann O, Bergsmann R. Projektionssymptome. 2nd ed. Vienna: Facultas; 1990.

Bischko J. Sonderformen der Akupunktur. Handbuch der Akupunktur und Aurikulotherapie [Brochure 21.4.0.]. Heidelberg: Haug; 1981.

Bischko J, ed. Weltkongress für wissenschaftliche Akupunktur [Proceedings of the World Congress for Scientific Acupuncture]. Part 1. Vienna, 1983.

Bischko J. Akupunktur für mäßig Fortgeschrittene. Vol. 2. 6th ed. Heidelberg: Haug; 1994.

Bischko J. Einführung in die Akupunktur. 16th ed. Heidelberg: Haug; 1997.

Gerhard I. Die Ohrakupunktur. Technik und Einsatz in der Gynäkologie sowie Ergebnis bei Sterilitätsbehandlung. Erfahrungsheilkunde. 1990;39:503–511.

Gerhard I, Müller C. Akupunktur in der Gynäkologie und Geburtshilfe. In: Dittmar, Loch, Wiesenauer, eds. Naturheilverfahren in der Frauenheilkunde und Geburtshilfe. 2nd ed. Stuttgart: Hippokrates; 1998.

Gerhard I, Postneek F. Auricular acupuncture in the treatment of female infertility. Obstet. Gynecol. 1987;69:57–60.

Gerhard I, Postneek F. Auricular acupuncture in the treatment of female infertility. Gynecologie and Endocrinology 1992 (6):171–181.

Gleditsch JM. Reflexzonen und Somatotopien als Schlüssel zu einer Gesamtschau des Menschen. 3rd ed. Schorndorf: WBV Biologisch-Medizinische Verlagsgesellschaft; 1988.

Gleditsch JM. MAPS–MikroAkuPunktSysteme. Stuttgart: Hippokrates; 2003.

Hecker H-U. VISDAK, Visuell-didaktisches System – eine kombinierte Darstellung von Bild und Text auf dem Gebiet der Akupunktur und Naturheilkunde. Application, German patent office Munich, 1997.

Hecker H-U, Steveling A. Die Akupunkturpunkte. 2nd ed. Stuttgart: Hippokrates; 2000.

Hecker H-U, Steveling A, Peuker ET, Kastner J, Liebchen K. Color Atlas of Acupuncture. Body Points, Ear Points, Trigger Points. Stuttgart–New York: Thieme; 2001.

Hecker H-U, Steveling A, Peuker ET, Kastner J. Practice of Acupuncture, Point Location – Treatment Options – TCM Basics. Stuttgart–New York: Thieme; 2004.

Helms JM. Acupuncture for the management of primary dysmenorrhea. Obstet. Gynecol. 1987;69:51–56.

Helms JM. Acupuncture Energetics. A clinical Approach for Physicians. Stuttgart-New York: Thieme; 2005.

Jacob E. Yamamoto's Scalp Acupuncture Seminar: A Presentation of Innovative Skills. J Altern Complement Med, Feb 2004;10(1):187–88.

Janda V. Manuelle Muskelfunktionsdiagnostik. 3rd ed. Berlin: Ullstein-Mosby; 1994.

Junghanns K-H. Akupunktur in der Geburtshilfe und Gynäkologie – Bereicherung der Therapiemöglichkeiten. Therapiewoche. 1992;43, 50: 2715–2720.

Junghanns K-H. Akupunktur in der Geburtshilfe und Frauenheilkunde – ein Naturheilverfahren als »sanfte Alternative«. Erfahrungsheilkunde. 1993;3:114–123.

Junghanns K-H. Akupunktur in der Geburtshilfe – Behandlungsmöglichkeiten am Beispiel der Ohrakupunktur. Gynäkol. Praxis. 1997:434–450.

Kendall F, Kendall E. Muscles – Testing and Function. 3rd ed. Baltimore: Williams & Wilkins; 1983.

König G, Wancura I. Praxis und Theorie der Neuen chinesischen Akupunktur. Vols. 1 and 2. Vienna: Maudrich; 1979/1983.

König G, Wancura I. Neue chinesische Akupunktur. Vienna: Maudrich; 1985.

König G, Wancura I. Einführung in die chinesische Ohrakupunktur. 9th ed. Heidelberg: Haug; 1989.

Kropeij H. Systematik der Ohrakupunktur. 7th ed. Heidelberg: Haug; 1993.

Lange G. Akupunktur in der Ohrmuschel, Diagnostik und Therapie. Schorndorf: WBV Biologisch-Medizinische Verlagsgesellschaft; 1985.

Lipton DS, Brewington, V, Smith, M. Acupuncture for crack-cocaine detoxification: experimental evaluation of efficacy. J Subst Abuse Treat. 1994 May–June;11(3):205–15.

Maciocia G. The Foundations of Chinese Medicine. New York: Churchill Livingston; 1989.

Marx H-G. Medikamentfreie Entgiftung von Suchtkranken – Bericht über den Einsatz der Akupunktur. Suchtgefahren. 1984;30.

Nogier P-M. From Auriculotherapy to Auriculomedicine. Saint-Ruffine: Maisonneuve; 1983.

Ogal HP, Hafer J, Ogal M, Krumholz W, Herget HF, Hempelmann G. Variations of pain in the treatment of one classical acupuncture point versus one point of Yamamoto's new scalp acupuncture. Anesthesiol Intensivmed Notfallmed Schmerzthr. 2002 June;37(6):326–32

Park JW. Su Jok (Hand & Foot) Acupuncture (Su Jok Acupuncture Series). Distributed by Korea Su Jok Acupuncture Institute; 1987.

Peuker ET, Filler TJ. The nerve supply of the human auricle. Clinical Anatomy. 2002;15:35–37.

Pothmann R, ed. Akupunktur-Repetitorum. 3rd ed. Stuttgart: Hippokrates; 1997.

Römer AT. Medical Acupuncture in Pregnancy. Stuttgart-New York: Thieme; 2005.

Römer AT, Seybold B. Akupunktur & TCM für die gynäkologische Praxis. Stuttgart: Hippokrates; 2001.

Rubach A. Principles of Ear Acupuncture – Microsystems of the Auricle. Stuttgart: Thieme; 2001.

Strauß K, Weidig W, eds. Akupunktur in der Suchtmedizin. 2nd ed. Stuttgart: Hippokrates; 1999.

Strittmatter B. Lokalisation der übergeordneten Punkte auf der Ohrmuschel. In: Der Akupunkturarzt/Aurikulotherapeut. Munich: Deutsche Akademie für Akupunktur und Aurikulomedizin e.V.; 1993.

Strittmatter B. Pocket Atlas of Ear Acupuncture. Stuttgart: Thieme; 2002.

Strittmatter B. Identifying and Treating Blockages to Healing. Stuttgart: Thieme; 2003.

Stux G, Berman B, Pomeranz B. Basics of Acupuncture. 5th ed. Berlin–Heidelberg–New York: Springer; 2003.

Travell JG, Simons DG. Myofacial Pain and Dysfunction, Vols 1 und 2. Baltimore: Williams & Wilkins; 1992.

Umlauf R. Zu den wissenschaftlichen Grundlagen der Aurikulotherapie. Dtsch. Z. Akupunktur. 1989;3:59–65.

Wiseman N, Feng Y. Practical Dictionary of Chinese Medicine. 2nd ed. Brookline, Mass.: Paradigm Publications; 1998.

Wühr E. Quintessenz der chinesischen Akupunktur und Moxibustion. Lehrbuch der chinesischen Hochschule für Traditionelle Chinesische Medizin. Kötzting: Verlag für Ganzheitliche Medizin, Dr. E. Wühr; 1988.

Yamamoto T, Yamamoto H: Yamamoto New Scalp Acupuncture. YNSA. Springer Japan; 1998.

Appendix

Index